THE
PARA
FITNESS
GUIDE

THE PARA FITNESS GUIDE

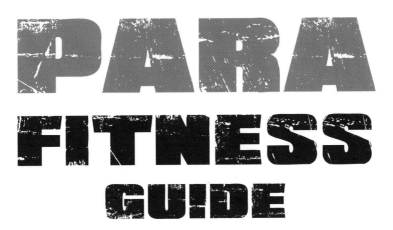

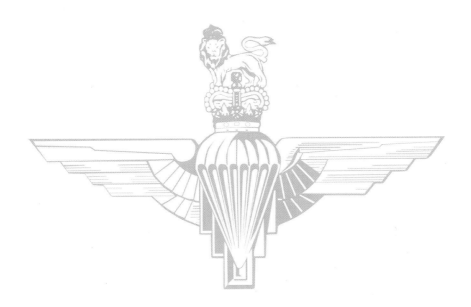

MAJOR SAM McGRATH

First published in Great Britain in 2010 by Osprey Publishing,
Midland House, West Way, Botley, Oxford OX2 OPH, United Kingdom.
44-02 23rd St, Suite 219, Long Island City, NY 11101, USA.

Email: info@ospreypublishing.com

A CIP catalogue record for this book is available from the British Library.

ISBN: 978 1 84908 546 5

Page layout by Myriam Bell Design, France
Typeset in Conduit and Univers Condensed
Originated by PDQ Digital Media Solutions, Suffolk, UK
Printed in Malta by Gutenberg Press Ltd.

11 12 13 14 15   10 9 8 7 6 5 4 3 2

EDITOR'S NOTE

CONVERSION TABLE
The following data will help in comparing the imperial and metric measurements:
1 mile = 1.6km
1 yard = 0.9m
1ft = 0.3m
1in. = 2.54cm/25.4mm
1 ton (US) = 0.9 tonnes
1lb = 0.45kg
1 gal = 4.5 liters

DISCLAIMER

If you are in any doubt whatsoever, you are strongly advised to
consult your physician before undertaking any of the activities
described in this book. Failure to do so may result in serious injury.
The Publisher and the Author will not accept any liability.

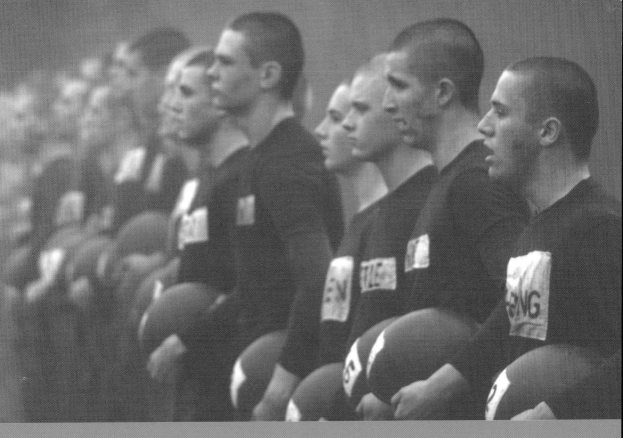

GET READY FOR ANYTHING...

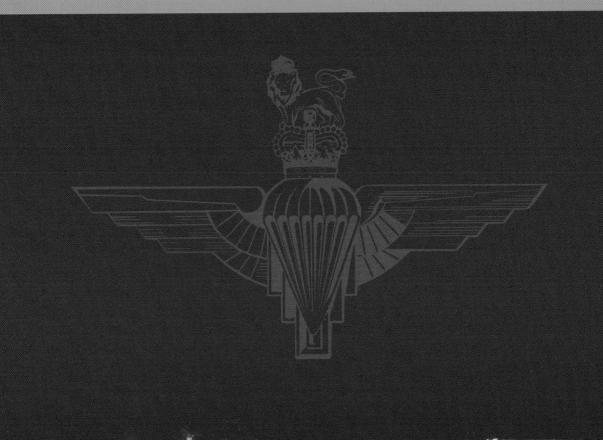

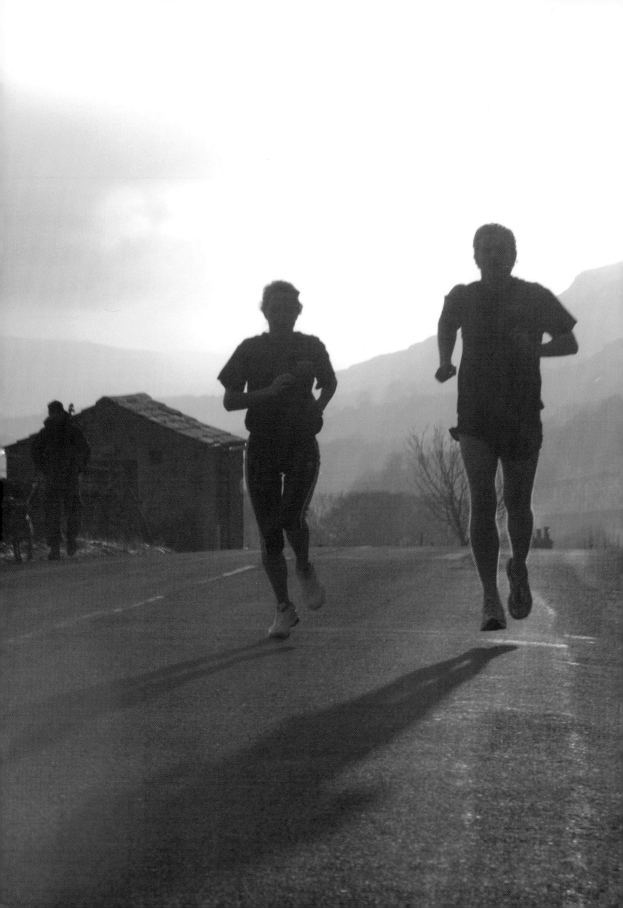

Dedication

For my beautiful daughter Eliza.

Acknowledgements

Throughout this project, I have relied heavily on the expertise and advice of Staff Sergeant Gavin Kirk, particularly on the more technical aspects of fitness program design. Gavin served as the Physical Training Instructor at P Company during for the first 18 months of my time as Officer Commanding. As paratrooper and physical training instructor he counts amongst the best I have had the pleasure of working with and I would not have been able to complete this book without his help. Thank you.

Thanks also to:

P Company and Para Company Staff, in particular Sergeant Majors Dickie Anderson and Steve Rayner for their support both on this project and during my tenure as OC P Company.

Lieutenant Colonel Paul Rodgers, Regimental Secretary The Parachute Regiment, for giving this book the Regiment's endorsement.

The MoD Press Office – in particular Paula Edwards and Sonja Hall.

Matt Timbers (www.matttimbers.com) and Channelle Knapp (www.elegance-photography) who provided the majority of the photographs used in this volume.

Grateful thanks also to Mrs Lorena Budd for her permission to use a photograph of her late husband Corporal Bryan Budd VC.

All royalties from the British sales of this book will go to Fairbridge and the Parachute Regiment Afghanistan Trust.

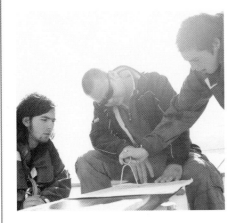

Fairbridge works with young people aged 13–25 that other organizations find difficult to engage – giving them the motivation, self-confidence and skills they need to change their lives.

Inside every disadvantaged young person, there is a confident, positive, individual trying to break out. Last year, Fairbridge helped 4,000 take their first step. Most were classed as having 'multiple needs', such as homelessness, substance misuse or a history of offending. Yet over the last 12 months, almost two-thirds went on to achieve something tangible. They returned to the classroom, started a college course, got a qualification or found a job. For these young people, Fairbridge was a new start – a chance to show the world who they really are.

Fairbridge worked.

Visit **www.fairbridge.org.uk** to find out more.

The Afghanistan Trust was formed in 2007 to help support soldiers and their families who have served with the Parachute Regiment in Afghanistan and who have been wounded or killed as a consequence.

A key part of which is purchasing mobility vehicles, car adaptations, wheel chairs and various life changing equipment which enable the servicean/woman to maintain a relatively normal lifestyle.

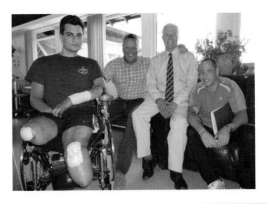

CONTENTS

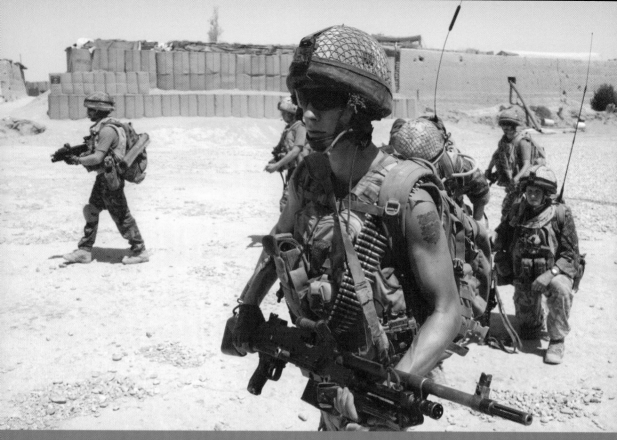

'WHAT MANNER OF MEN ARE THESE THAT WEAR THE MAROON BERET?'

'They are firstly all volunteers and are toughened by physical training.
As a result they have infectious optimism and that offensive eagerness
which comes from physical well-being. They have jumped from the air and
by doing so have conquered fear.

Their duty lies in the van of the battle. They are proud of their honour and
have never failed at any task. They have the highest standards in all things
whether it be skill in battle or smartness in the execution of all peacetime
duties. They are, in fact, men apart – every man an emperor.

Of all the factors which make for success in battle, the spirit of the warrior
is the most decisive. That spirit will be found in full measure in the men
who wear the maroon beret.'

Field Marshal Viscount Montgomery of Alamein

INTRODUCTION

Welcome to my guide to how to become PARA fit. Whether your goal is to row the Atlantic, lose weight for health reasons or something in-between, this book has everything you need. It details a tried and tested fitness recipe that will not only help you improve your health and fitness, but also your confidence and motivation. Twelve years ago I joined the British Parachute Regiment, more commonly known as the 'PARAS', because I wanted to serve with the best and achieve my potential. Today my aim is to give you the tools to achieve your potential too.

Fitness and the PARAS have been my passions for most of my life. While at school my one goal was to win my maroon beret, and that aim remained my focus throughout my teenage years. I accomplished it on my first attempt, shortly after my 19th birthday. And as the Officer Commanding P (Pegasus) Company, my job was to ensure that the next generation of paratroopers lived up to the exacting standards of the PARAS. For two years, the responsibility for training and selecting all British Army paratroopers sat on my shoulders. The privilege of training and fighting alongside thousands of PARAS has given me a unique insight into what it is that makes our regiment special. Our soldiers are undoubtedly the building blocks, but I believe the glue that binds us together is the confidence and motivation which comes from acquiring supreme physical fitness.

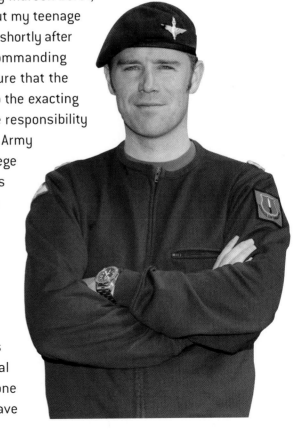

The PARAS are a team that succeeds because of our mental and physical toughness and our commitment to one another. Since our creation in 1942, we have

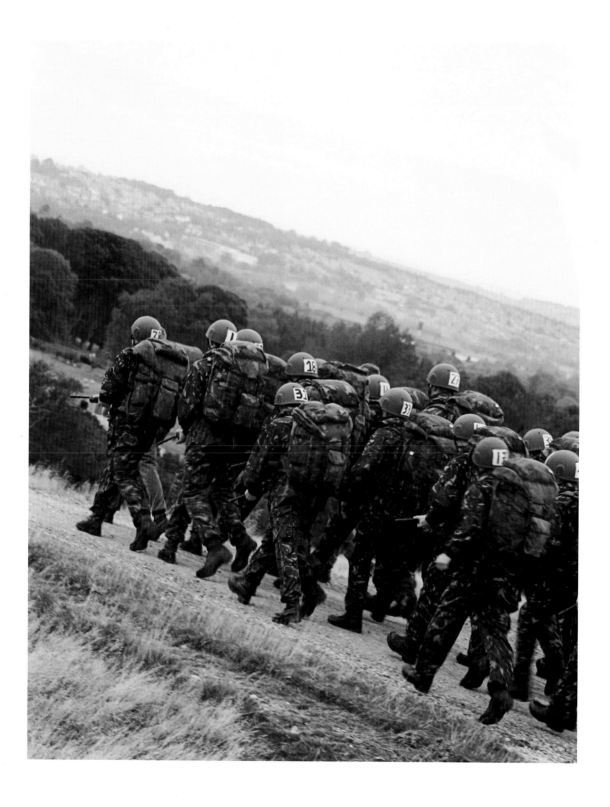

refined a training and selection process which turns young school-leavers into paratroopers – arguably among the fittest and most intimidating soldiers in the world. While much of PARA training concerns technical and tactical skills, by far the most important part is training our recruits to achieve things they didn't consider possible. Through a progressive physical fitness training programme we not only produce superb warriors, but also instil a confidence, pride and mental fortitude that has relevance beyond the gym, aerobics studio and athletics track. All of this results in paratroopers who are ready for anything...

Inspired by the PARA training programme, this book offers two different approaches to achieving your goal. The first (the Spartan Programme) closely follows the types of activities we use to make paratroopers, and requires little more than a watch and a pair of trainers. The second (the Emperor Programme), while potentially just as demanding, incorporates some modern-day luxuries. While facts tell, stories sell, so as a source of inspiration I have included in this book accounts of PARA missions which I believe capture the essence of what physical fitness and the PARA mindset are all about.

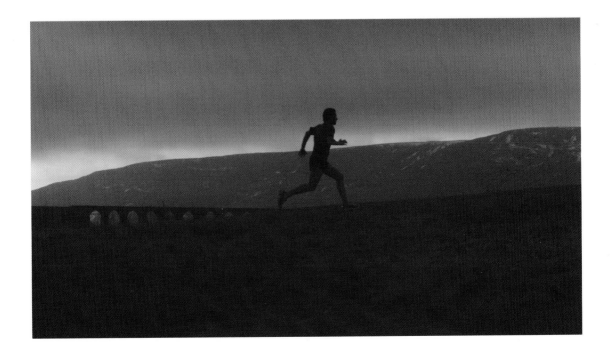

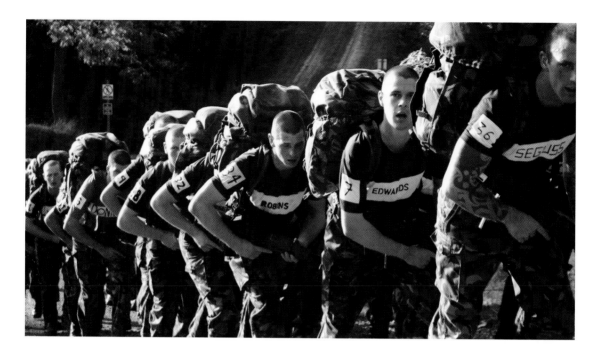

Along with the unique content of the PARA programme, what separates this book from other fitness books is that I live what I preach. As a Parachute Regiment commander I intimately understand motivation, both as a performance athlete and as an instructor. Throughout the next eight weeks I will impart the knowledge and skills to help you define your goal, recognize its significance and then devise your most effective means of achieving it. However, in just five weeks, this training programme has the potential to change your life forever. Whether fighting a fierce enemy or a sedentary lifestyle, second place equals defeat and an early death. In the PARAS winning is everything – in this book your body is our battlefield.

Major Sam McGrath

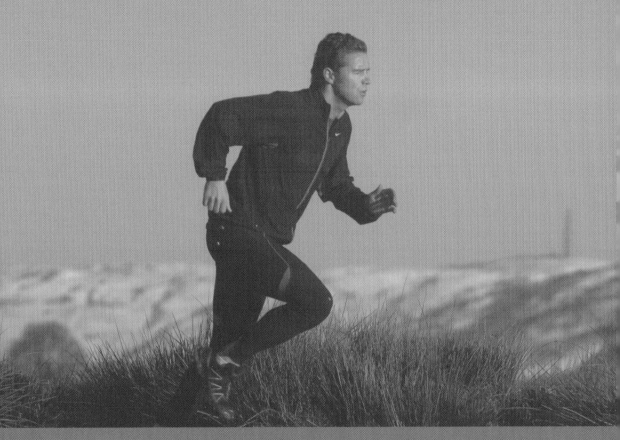

PART 1:
READY FOR ANYTHING

Utrinque Paratus

Regimental motto of the Parachute Regiment – 'Ready for Anything'

The PARAS - Train Hard, Fight Easy

Military parachuting remains one of the most difficult and important military tasks undertaken today. Parachute operations use shock tactics which seek to surprise the enemy in order to achieve a swift victory. For the United Kingdom, the PARAS are a 'break glass in case of emergency' organization; a force that enables our country to respond immediately and decisively to a crisis, wherever it is.

Paratroopers, unlike conventional soldiers, must be capable of overcoming a superior number of enemy troops armed only with the equipment they carry on their backs. Resupply is often only available by air, typically at least 48 hours after insertion due to the threat posed by enemy aircraft. In order to maximize the availability of equipment

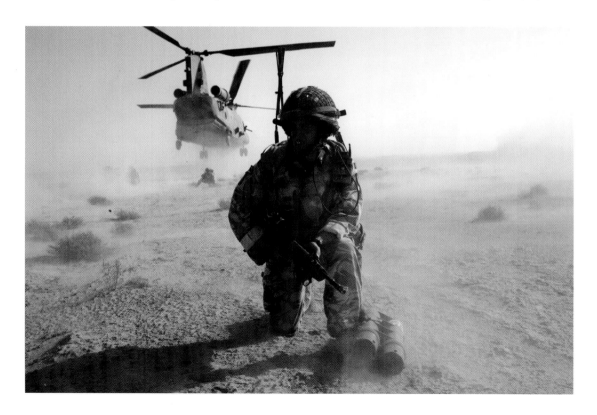

and ammunition each paratrooper is loaded to the capacity of their parachute; their rucksacks often weigh more than they do.

Uncertainty and anxiety surrounds every aspect of a parachute operation. Planned in secret, each operation starts with weeks of exhaustive planning and rehearsal, frequently based on scarce intelligence. Air insertions on RAF C-130 Hercules aircraft are long and uncomfortable. Low-level flying and hot, stuffy conditions guarantee that no one sleeps and almost everyone is sick; these conditions could have been purposely designed to degrade the passengers. By the time PARAS have reached their destination, the fear of jumping is quickly overcome by a desire to get out of the flying hellhole.

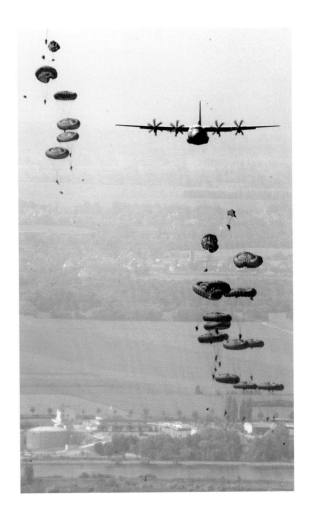

Drop Zones (DZ) are selected roughly ten miles away from enemy objectives, a distance chosen to balance surprise with the need to avoid enemy air defences as the PARAS are most vulnerable when jumping. The DZ is a scene of utter confusion. Terrain, weather and the enemy almost certainly guarantee that paratroopers either don't reach the DZ or land in the wrong place. The chaos of the DZ demands *ad hoc* planning and regrouping at every level. Soldiers and resources must be continually reallocated in accordance with changing priorities, often in the face of enemy fire.

From the DZ the PARAS conduct a Tactical Advance to Battle (TAB). The TAB is normally a ten-mile forced march, the aim of which is to deliver the PARAS and all their kit to their objective in under two hours, before the enemy has had time to prepare its defence. What follows is a fight for survival.

For the PARAS fitness is not an end in itself. It is a necessity which enables us to cope with the unique demands of our role. However, fitness only captures a small part of the demands placed on paratroopers. By the time a paratrooper faces his enemy, he has had to overcome numerous mental and physical obstacles that dilute his fighting ability: scant intelligence, a tortuous flight and parachute descent, and a gruelling insertion march carrying the equivalent of his own body weight. This type of soldiering requires a resilience and flexibility of mind unlike any other.

For the UK the primary response to an overseas crisis is fulfilled by 16 Air Assault Brigade's Lead Airborne Task Force. Spearheaded by the Parachute Regiment, the force comprises a battle group of nearly 1,200 paratroopers. It is capable of deploying anywhere in the world, to conduct any type of military task, within 24 hours. It is for this reason that the PARAS train and select soldiers using standards above and beyond those of the rest of the army. However, although many are called to try for the chance to serve with the PARAS, few are chosen.

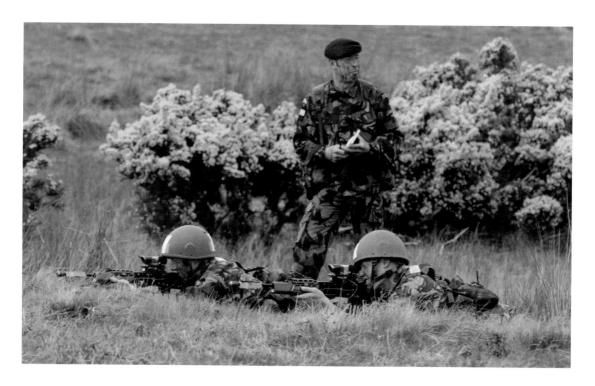

Paratrooper Training

The process of joining the PARAS is long and tortuous. All soldiers, including officers, who wish to serve with airborne forces must first pass Pre-Parachute Selection. Pegasus (P) Company, the organization responsible for running this selection, consists of 12 hand-picked instructors who serve as the custodians of airborne standards. The P Company mission is:

To test the physical fitness, determination and mental robustness, under conditions of stress, to determine whether an individual has the self-discipline and motivation required for service with Airborne Forces.

The common high standards attained by PARA recruits are fundamental to the ethos of airborne forces. By design, P Company takes students beyond their own appetite for challenge, testing their physical and mental robustness, and in doing so assesses their commitment and suitability for parachute operations. The prize, for those who are successful, is the award of the coveted maroon beret and the opportunity to go on to take the Basic Parachute Course at RAF Brize Norton.

TEST WEEK

Test Week is the culmination of P Company training. Parachute Regiment recruits attempt Test Week in the latter stages of their Combined Infantry Course (CIC) in their first few months in the army. Serving soldiers are also eligible to attempt to join the PARAS, but they must pass the longer All Arms P Company course, where Test Week follows a two-and-a-half-week 'build-up' phase. The Territorial Army (TA) recruits attend a condensed four-day Pre-Parachute Selection course preceded by eight months of fitness and military training.

Test Week comprises eight separate events over a four-and-a-half day period. Seven events are scored out of ten. However, all must pass the

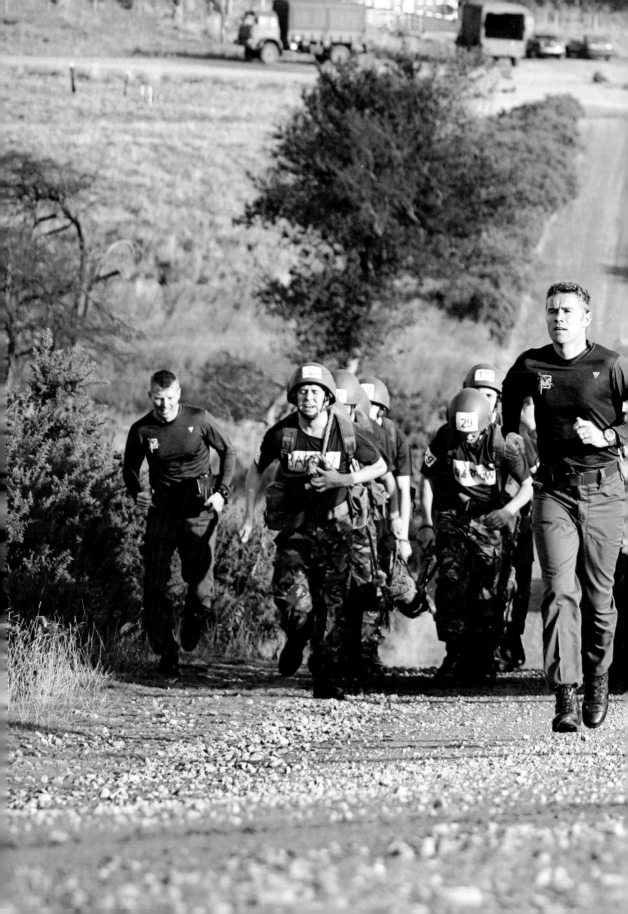

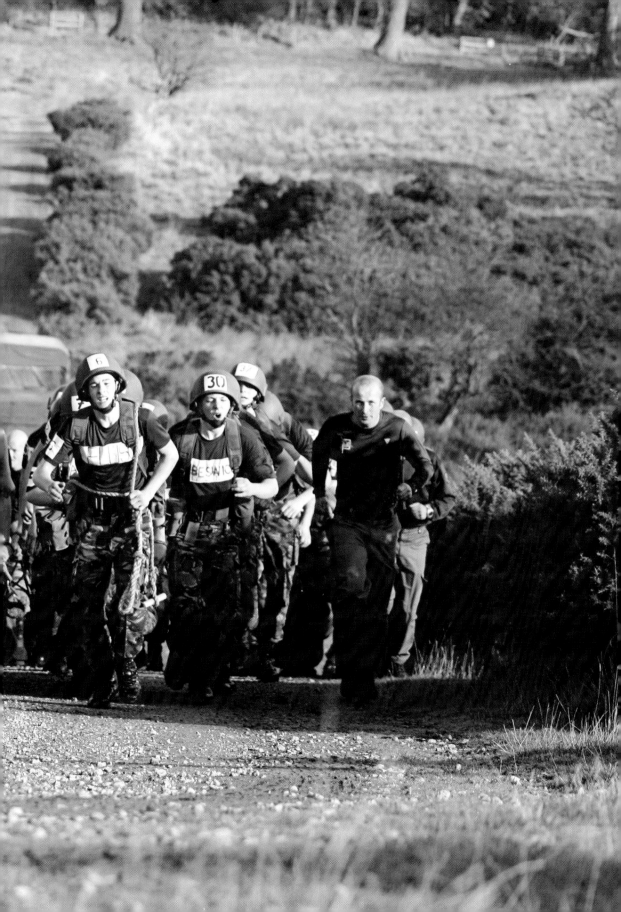

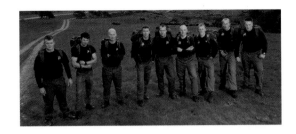

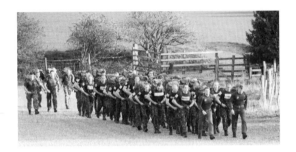

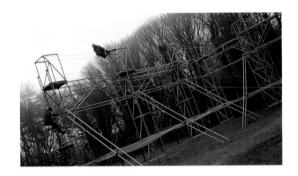

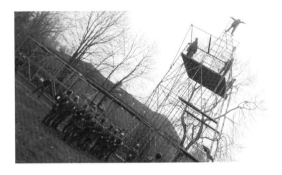

From top: P Company staff, the ten mile-march and the Trainasium. The Trainasium includes such simple tests as bending to touch your toes – but at the highest point of a 55ft structure.

Trainasium event. Candidates must score a total of 45 points to pass. Points are awarded in accordance with the P Company Charter, a document that ensures the consistency of the tests and the validity of the selection. Each event is designed to assess a candidate's physical fitness, mental robustness and determination. A candidate who fails to display the appropriate level of self-discipline and motivation throughout Test Week will fail the course. Test Week starts on a Wednesday morning and finishes the following Tuesday. The tests are as follows:

TEN-MILE MARCH (WEDNESDAY MORNING)

The ten-mile march is conducted as a squad, over undulating terrain, with each candidate carrying a Bergen (backpack) weighing 35lbs (plus water) and a rifle. The march must be completed in less than one hour and 50 minutes. TA candidates have two hours. This event was the inspiration behind the PARAS' 10 endurance race (www.paras10.com) which I revived in 2008 and features in Part 7.

TRAINASIUM (WEDNESDAY AFTERNOON)

The Trainasium is a superb 'Aerial Confidence Course' which is unique to P Company. It is used to assess and train candidates for military parachuting, specifically by testing their ability to overcome fear and carry out simple activities and instructions at heights up to 55ft.

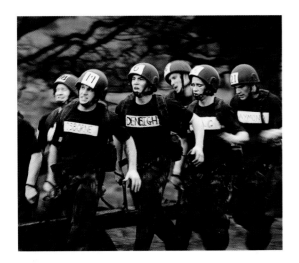

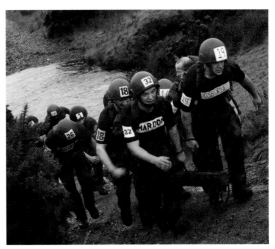

LOG RACE (THURSDAY MORNING)

During the Log Race teams of eight, carrying a 132lb log, must complete a harrowing 1.9-mile course as quickly as possible — typically within 15 minutes. This event stains each candidate's soul; to this day it remains the hardest physical challenge I have ever encountered.

The Log Race – with a log the size of a telegraph pole over difficult, hilly terrain.

STEEPLECHASE (THURSDAY AFTERNOON)

This individual race over a demanding 1.8-mile, cross-country course, includes a number of 'water obstacles' and an assault course. Candidates must complete the event in under 19 minutes to score ten points.

Steeplechasing through water and over obstacles.

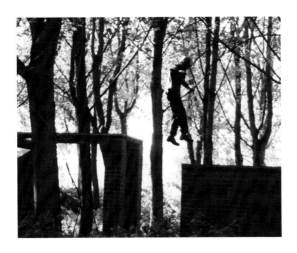

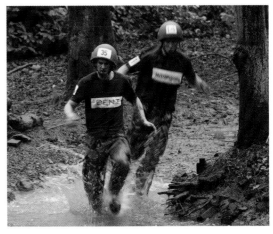

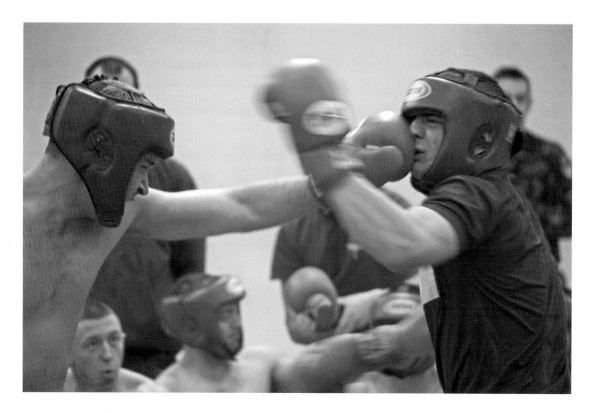

Milling is used to simulate the stress of a soldier's first combat experience.

TWO-MILE MARCH (FRIDAY MORNING)

This is an individual, best-effort event, where each candidate has 18 minutes to complete an undulating two-mile course carrying a 35lb Bergen.

MILLING (FRIDAY AFTERNOON)

This 60 seconds of 'controlled physical aggression' against an opponent of similar height and weight simulates the mental stress encountered during a soldier's first contact (gun battle). The combination of neither wishing to be hurt nor perform badly amongst peers makes the physical aspects of the event all the more difficult.

ENDURANCE MARCH (MONDAY)

Conducted as a squad, with each member carrying a 35lb Bergen, this 20-mile march over the hills of the Yorkshire Dales has to be completed in less than four hours and 10 minutes.

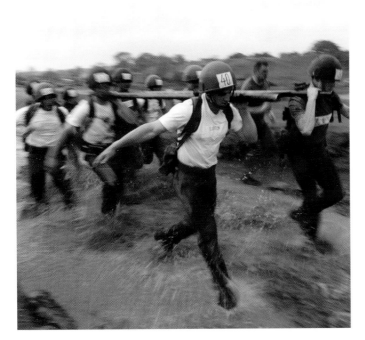

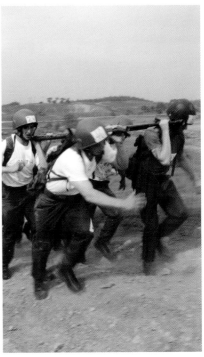

STRETCHER RACE (TUESDAY MORNING)

This is the final event of Test Week. Teams of 12 men take turns to carry a 175lb stretcher over a distance of five miles. No more than four men carry the stretcher at any given time. Participants wear webbing and carry a rifle.

The Stretcher Race tests endurance, with the course including hills and rough terrain. It is often considered the most arduous of all the tests.

Unlike other elite military physical selection courses, such as the Royal Marines Commando course or SAS hills selection, P Company students receive no feedback on their performance during Test Week. This lack of information makes the selection much more difficult, because students spend their entire week second-guessing and worrying about whether a pass is still attainable. It is for this reason that the majority of failures during Test Week come from those voluntarily withdrawing (VW) themselves from the course. At the end of P Company, those who pass have not only proved that they have the physical qualities of a paratrooper, but that they are able to cope with the mental stress — which on the battlefield is every bit as important.

Fit to Fight, Fit for Life

The PARAS have an approach to preparing soldiers for the battlefield which typifies our state of mind. It is captured perfectly by the P Company mantra, 'if you train hard, you fight easy'. Experience has shown us that supreme physical fitness results in soldiers who are physically and psychologically better conditioned to deal with the various stresses of the modern battlefield. Not only are our soldiers physically more resilient, but they have greater confidence and motivation which enables them to perform better when tired or under stress.

Collectively, this method of carefully training and selecting personnel results in an organization that enjoys a unique sense of collective identity and camaraderie, built on mutual trust and confidence in one another. You may have experienced this kind of closeness in great teams you have been a part of. On the battlefield, fear is your greatest enemy, but we have learnt to use this to our advantage. Our train hard, fight easy approach gives us a decisive edge; we expect and plan for success while letting our enemies defeat themselves, intimidated by our reputation.

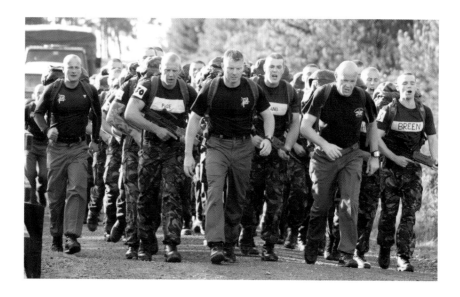

While there are many physical jobs and vocations in the world, the PARAS sit at an extreme edge. Few professions require their people to be capable of enduring extreme situations that are both physically and mentally degrading, before having to overcome a superior enemy armed only with surprise and determination. However, regardless of how active your job is, science has proved that being in good physical shape can significantly enhance the quality of your life. Therefore, a good physical fitness regime can be truly transformational.

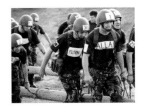

There is overwhelming scientific research to support the fact that people who lead active lifestyles are less likely to suffer from illness and are more likely to live longer. Some of the health benefits of exercise are described here.

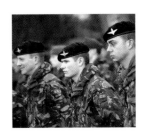

HEART & CIRCULATORY SYSTEM

- Exercise halves your risk of heart disease and stroke, one of the greatest causes of illness and death.
- Doing exercise can reduce high blood pressure (hypertension).
- Exercise can reduce your ('harmful') high-density lipoprotein (HDL) cholesterol.
- Regular physical activity can help fend off, or help manage, Type 2 diabetes by controlling your blood sugar levels. Poorly controlled blood sugar levels can damage your eyes, nerves, kidneys and arteries.

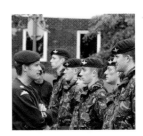

SKELETAL SYSTEM

- Eight out of ten people have joint or lower back pain at some time in their lives. However, people who exercise are less likely to suffer from it.
- Osteoporosis (when your bones become brittle and prone to fracture) can be delayed, or controlled, by exercise. High-impact exercise, such as running, increases bone density and slows down bone degeneration later in life. Low-impact exercise, such as gentle walking or swimming, can help those already suffering from osteoporosis.

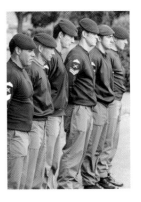

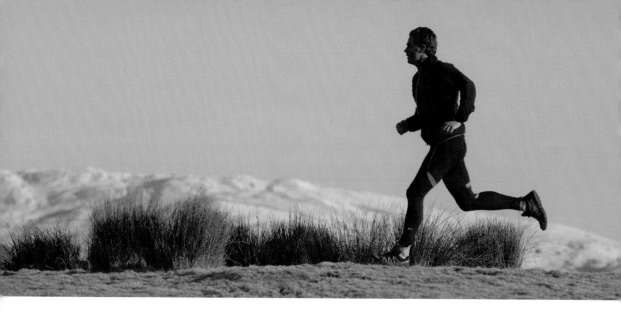

CANCER

- You are less likely to develop cancer if you are physically active.
- Research has shown that exercise protects against colon cancer and against breast cancer in women who have been through the menopause. This research is complemented by studies that suggest exercise may also help prevent lung and endometrial cancers.

WEIGHT MANAGEMENT & GENERAL HEALTH

- Excess calories are stored as fat, so you put on weight when you eat more calories than you use. Physical activity uses calories and so helps to create a healthy energy balance. Physical activity alone can help you lose weight if you are overweight or obese – the more you do, the more weight you will lose. However, combining exercise with a healthy diet will mean you lose weight faster.
- Obesity (excessive weight, caused by an imbalance between your energy intake from food and energy output through activity) doubles your risk of heart disease, stroke and Type 2 diabetes. It also increases the possibility that you will develop joint problems and some cancers.

Although we've heard about the significant health benefits of an active lifestyle, personally I believe the psychological gains that come from getting and staying fit are even more beneficial. Fear and anxiety are not restricted to the battlefield, just as confidence, motivation and the ability to deal with stress are as relevant to your success as a student, parent, professional or athlete as they are to a paratrooper.

Extensive research has proved that exercise not only makes you physically fitter, it also improves your mental health and general sense of well-being. When you look good, you feel better, but the impact of staying fit is much greater than this:

- Exercise can have a positive effect on those at risk from mental illnesses. Leading an inactive lifestyle for long periods of time means you are more likely to suffer from clinical depression. Some studies suggest that regular exercise can be as effective as talking treatments or medicines in the management of depression, while having fewer side-effects.
- You may also benefit from exercise if you have anxiety-related disorders, such as phobias, panic attacks or stress.
- You are likely to feel happier, more satisfied with life and have an improved sense of well-being if you are physically active. Introduce regular exercise into your routine and you should sleep better, lower your stress levels and boost your self-image. It is also possible that it may improve brain function in children and older adults.

So now that you know the overwhelming physical and mental health benefits that come from an active lifestyle, let's begin the transformation and get you in paratrooper shape!

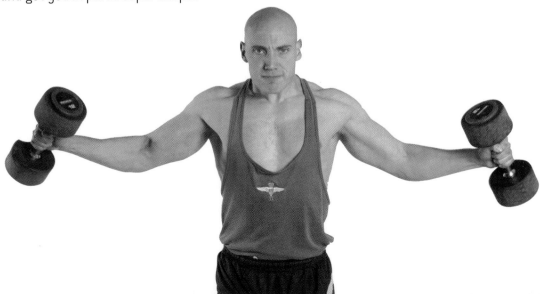

CORPORAL BRYAN BUDD, VICTORIA CROSS
'Strength of mind, strength of cause'

Corporal Bryan Budd VC stands for everything the Parachute Regiment was built on. While perhaps an unusual example to use, I believe the citation of Corporal Budd's gallantry medal illustrates perfectly the human capacity to absorb extreme mental and physical anxiety in the pursuit of a goal – in this instance the preservation of the lives of his men.

Corporal Budd joined the Parachute Regiment in December 1995 and spent the majority of his time with the Pathfinder Platoon, an elite group within the PARAS which performs all advance force operations for 16 Air Assault Brigade. (A description of one of the Pathfinder Platoon selection tests, the Fan Dance, is included in Part 7.) He was posted to A Company of 3 PARA in early June 2006 in the middle of Operation *Herrick IV*, serving in Helmand Province at a time when the company was principally concerned with helping the Afghan government to counter the resurgence in Taliban activity centred in and around the town of Sangin. During July and August 2006, A Company, 3rd Battalion the Parachute Regiment was deployed in the District Centre at Sangin. It constantly came under sustained attack from a combination of Taliban small arms, rocket-propelled grenade, mortar and rocket fire.

> *On 27 July 2006, whilst on a routine patrol, Corporal Bryan Budd's section identified and engaged two enemy gunmen on the roof of a building in the centre of Sangin. During the ensuing fierce fire-fight, two of Corporal*

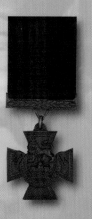

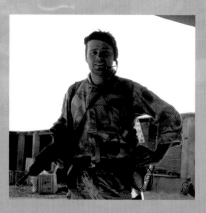

Budd's section were hit. One was seriously injured and collapsed in the open ground, where he remained exposed to enemy fire, with rounds striking the ground around him. Corporal Budd realised that he needed to regain the initiative and that the enemy needed to be driven back so that the casualty could be evacuated.

Under fire, he personally led the attack on the building where the enemy fire was heaviest, forcing the remaining fighters to flee across an open field where they were successfully engaged. This courageous and prompt action proved decisive in breaking the enemy and was undertaken at great personal risk. Corporal Budd's decisive leadership and conspicuous gallantry allowed his wounded colleague to be evacuated to safety where he subsequently received life-saving treatment.

A month later, on 20 August 2006, Corporal Budd was leading his section on the right forward flank of a platoon clearance patrol near Sangin District Centre. Another section was advancing with a Land Rover fitted with a .50 calibre heavy machine gun on the patrol's left flank. Pushing through thick vegetation, Corporal Budd identified a number of enemy fighters 30 metres ahead. Undetected, and in an attempt to surprise and destroy the enemy, Corporal Budd initiated a flanking manoeuvre. However, the enemy spotted the Land Rover on the left flank and the element of surprise was lost for the whole platoon.

In order to regain the initiative, Corporal Budd decided to assault the enemy and ordered his men to follow him. As they moved forward the section came under a withering fire that incapacitated three of his men. The continued enemy fire and these losses forced the section to take cover. But, Corporal Budd continued to assault on his own, knowing full well the likely consequences of doing so without the close support of his remaining men. He was wounded but continued to move forward, attacking and killing the enemy as he rushed their position.

Inspired by Corporal Budd's example, the rest of the platoon reorganized and pushed forward their attack, eliminating more of the enemy and eventually forcing their withdrawal. Corporal Budd subsequently died of his wounds, and when his body was later recovered it was found surrounded by three dead Taliban.

Corporal Budd's conspicuous gallantry during these two engagements saved the lives of many of his colleagues. He acted in the full knowledge that the rest of his men had either been struck down or had been forced to go to ground. His determination to press home a single-handed assault against a superior enemy force despite his wounds stands out as a premeditated act of inspirational leadership and supreme valour. In recognition of this, Corporal Budd is awarded the Victoria Cross.

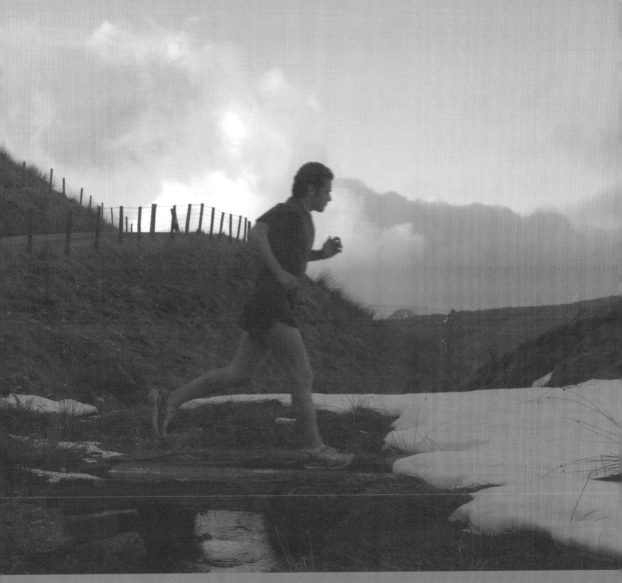

PART 2:
PRELIMINARY OPERATIONS

'What we obtain too cheap, we esteem too lightly; it is dearness only that gives everything its value.'
Thomas Paine

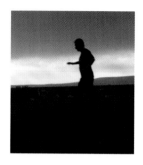

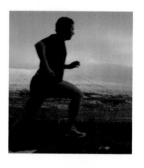

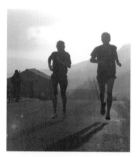

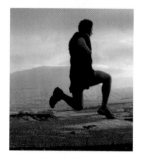

Before the Parachute Regiment conducts a mission, we undertake an intensive period of both mental and physical preparation. Like the two wheels of a bicycle, these two elements are equally important, and with either one missing the journey will be over before it has begun. The military is perhaps the only organization that specializes in conducting one-off, large-scale complex operations. Through a constant cycle of training and evaluating previous missions we have developed an exhaustive array of Standard Operating Procedures (SOPs) detailing everything from how we maintain our vehicle fleet to how we rally after a parachute jump or manoeuvre as a group in the assault. SOPs cover both individuals and large bodies of troops, providing a common way of dealing with situations so everyone instinctively knows how to conduct themselves in specific circumstances, and using lessons learnt from the past to make us more efficient and effective in the future. SOPs are tried and tested in a controlled environment as we incrementally condition ourselves to deal with the mental and physical hurdles between us and success. An example of this is that we learn how to shoot on the ranges first, before going through a series of gradual steps prior to being tasked to use a rifle on an operational mission. Our SOPs enable us to compress the time between being tasked with an objective and being able to execute it successfully.

A critical part of SOPs involves educating all involved in what we believe to be the best way of dealing with a particular scenario. By doing this, we ensure that every soldier is capable of assuming the role of their immediate commander, so that the loss of one man does not mean failure. In this chapter our focus is on fitness SOPs. These SOPs, like our mission SOPs, have evolved through experience, evaluation and constant review. However, the objective is not just that you understand what you should do before, during and after exercise, but why you should do it. By developing this understanding you will not only be more committed to following these principles, but you will be able to gain the confidence and knowledge to develop your own programme tailored to your specific exercise goals.

Physical Preparation

I want you to think of your new fitness regime as a journey. Before you set off on any journey it's critical to know where you're starting from. This is because your starting point not only tells you which direction to go in, but during the journey it enables you to measure how far you've come and how far you have left to go.

For a potential PARA the starting point of the transition from Clark Kent to Superman is his fitness level on Day One of basic training. To use the Superman metaphor a little longer, there's a combination of factors which make Clark Kent capable of being Superman, some of them genetic, some of them environmental. Potential PARAS are no different. We identify our Clark Kents by using two simple but stringent checks: a fitness test and a medical examination. No one gets past Day One without passing both.

In the medical examination we are ensuring that Private Kent has no serious ailments that might prevent him from fulfilling the role of a paratrooper. In the fitness test we're establishing a common start point which we can build on. As Private Kent's destination requires an awe-inspiring level of fitness and we have only a fixed amount of time (19 weeks) to get him there, entry requirements are high: ten overarm pull-ups; over 60 sit-ups in 2 minutes; over 80 press-ups in two minutes; followed by completing a 1½-mile run in under nine minutes 18 seconds. (It is worth noting that the Parachute Regiment's required fitness standard at the start of training is higher than that of the rest of the British Army at the *end* of their basic training.) Before we set about transforming you into superman or superwoman, we need to establish where we're starting from.

MEDICAL FITNESS

At the very start of this book is a warning to seek medical advice if you are in any doubt as to whether you are capable of starting a fitness regime. This is a point which is worth emphasizing. As a way of addressing any potential concerns, use the checklist below to decide whether you should seek medical advice:

- Have you had heart trouble?
- Do you frequently suffer from chest pain?
- Do you often feel faint or suffer from dizziness?
- Do you suffer from high blood pressure?
- Do you suffer from bone or joint problems that are aggravated by exercise?
- Is there is any other physical reason why you should not follow a physical activity programme?
- Are you over 65 and unaccustomed to vigorous exercise?
- Are you using drugs which might alter your response to exercise?

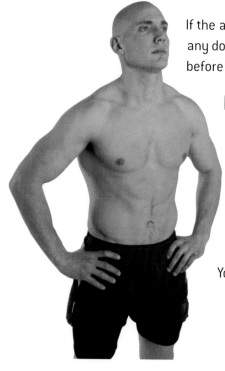

If the answer to any of the questions above is 'yes', or if you have any doubt whatsoever, then it is essential that you consult a doctor before you start exercising.

BODY MASS INDEX (BMI)

Your BMI is a simple and effective way of assessing whether you are at a healthy weight. Like many quick assessments the BMI has its limitations; for instance, in most cases a bodybuilder in peak fitness will be categorized as being overweight, or even obese, due to the density of his muscles.

$$\text{Your BMI} = \frac{(\text{your weight in kilograms / your height in metres})}{\text{your height in metres}}$$

Underweight	Lower than 18.5
Healthy weight	18.5–24.9
Overweight	25–29.9
Obese	30–39.9

HEART RATE

An easy way of assessing your general health is to check the number of beats your heart gives in a minute. Heart rate increases with age and lack of exercise. As a general rule the slower your heart rate, the fitter you are. You can check your heart rate by placing two fingers (not your thumb, which has its own pulse) on your carotid artery; this is on both sides of your neck, just next to your Adam's apple. Using a watch, count the number of times your heart beats in 15 seconds and multiply the result by four to get your heart rate. Your resting heart rate is best taken when you wake up, as you are then in your most relaxed state.

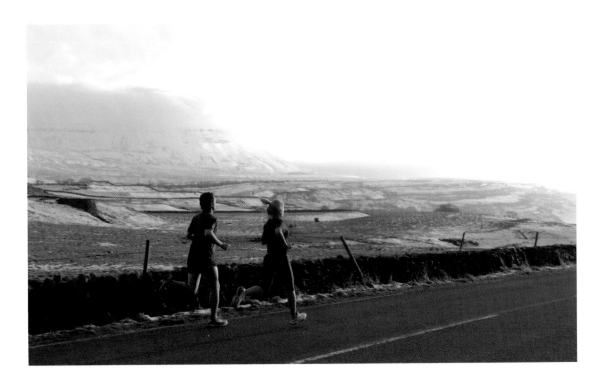

PHYSICAL FITNESS

There are many ways to assess your starting point, but this is a PARA fitness guide so we are going to use the entrance test used for all PARA recruits. Be sensible. If you need to abbreviate or adapt any of the tests, that's fine so long as you use the same test later on during your programme to assess your progress – consistency is the key. For those who feel they'll walk the test, prove it; we'll be ramping up the pace in no time with some more challenging fitness tests. However, this entrance test forms the foundations of your PARA programme.

THE PARA ENTRANCE FITNESS TEST

After performing the warm-up described in Part 4 on pages 83–92, perform as many of the PARA fitness test activities as you can, ensuring you include a two-minute break between each exercise. After each activity record the relevant data (number of repetitions, time or distance) and compare it with the table provided on page 40. The PARA entrance fitness test is a simple but effective test, which will show you your fitness level quickly and efficiently. With the exception of the pull-up test you should be able to do all individual tests in the immediate vicinity of your house.

STRENGTH & MUSCULAR ENDURANCE TESTS
Pull-up test

Pull-ups are an excellent test of your body to weight strength and, in my opinion, the most relevant measure of your strength. Complete as many pull-ups as you can without touching the floor or letting go of the bar. (For a complete explanation of the exercise, see Part 5, pages 111–113.) If you're not a member of a gym, finding an appropriate bar can be a struggle and in the past I've always used the monkey bars in a children's park. If you do not have access to a bar, then we can get by without doing this test.

Two-minute press-up test

The press-up is a fantastic measure of upper body muscular endurance. Perform as many press-ups as you can in two minutes, taking time to rest as appropriate within this time. (For a complete explanation of the exercise, see Part 5, pages 106–108.)

Two-minute sit-up test

The sit-up is a great test of trunk muscular endurance. Complete as many repetitions as you can in two minutes, resting when necessary. (For a complete explanation of the exercise, see Part 5, pages 114–116.)

CARDIOVASCULAR FITNESS TESTS
1½-mile/2.4km run

After walking and jogging for a ½ mile (the warm-up), complete 1½ miles in the quickest possible time. If you're unable to run the whole distance, jog or walk as is necessary. You can measure the distance either by running the distance on a treadmill, or by using an odometer on your car or bike to measure the distance before you run it. Alternatively, you can use a 400m running track and do two laps for the warm-up followed by six laps for the test.

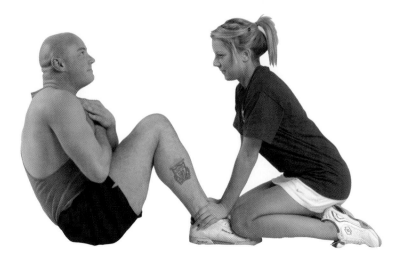

Flexibility

The sit-and-reach test is a test of flexibility in the lower back and hamstrings. As shown in the picture, sit facing a wall with your legs outstretched. Lean forwards, sliding your fingers along the floor towards the wall to a position that you can hold for at least five seconds — best marked using a 30cm ruler. Your score is the distance the between the ends of your fingers and the wall.

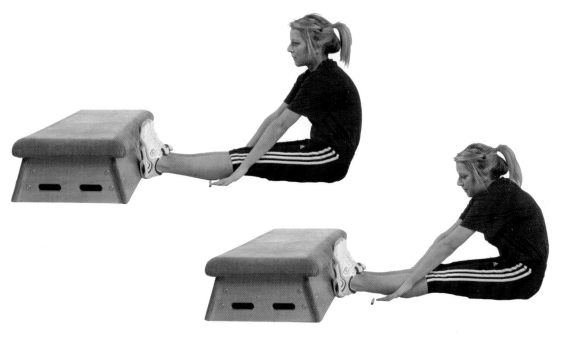

PERFORMANCE STANDARDS				
Activity	Civilian	Recruit	Soldier	Paratrooper
Pull-ups	0–5	6–10	11–17	18 or more
Press-ups (2 minutes)	0–29	30–49	50–79	80 or more
Sit-ups (2 minutes)	0–29	30–49	50–79	80 or more
1½-mile run	12min 31sec to 18min	10min 31sec to 12min 30sec	8min 1sec to 10min 30sec	Under 8min
Sit-and-reach test	60–31cm	30–21cm	11–20cm	Under 10cm
BMI	30–39.9	25–29.9	18.5–24.9	Under 18.5
Resting heart rate	80–110	65–80	50–65	Under 50

Planning the Attack

Whenever paratroopers are given a specific mission, they are not only told what they must achieve, but why they must achieve it. My experience is that paratroopers only truly commit to a plan when they believe it is worthwhile, the methodology is logical and they stand a high chance of success. Following this logic, before we embark on the PARA fitness programme I believe it is important that we understand what fitness is, how it can be improved and how certain types of exercise programme are more effective the others. This ultimately will give you the ability to write your own fitness programmes to achieve your specific goals, fitted around your lifestyle.

WHAT IS FITNESS?

Fitness is a relative concept – what one person may consider an extreme physical challenge, another may dismiss as a sedentary pastime. According to dictionary.com a definition of fit is: 'qualified, or suited to some purpose, function or situation'. Therefore, 'fitness' should be considered in relation to your capacity to meet the demands you are likely to place on your body during the course of your life. In the PARAS we measure physical fitness in relation to airborne soldiering. We assess this in our recruits during P Company and thereafter using various measures depending on what the specific PARA unit is required to do at a particular time.

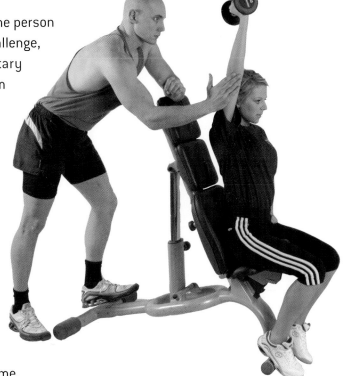

Fitness can be broken down into four components: endurance, strength, speed and flexibility.

Endurance

Endurance comes in two main forms – aerobic endurance and muscular endurance. Aerobic endurance is the term given to the capacity of your heart and lungs to send oxygen to your muscles in order to sustain a specific level of activity, e.g. running. Muscular endurance refers to the capacity of a muscle, or muscle group, to perform repeated contractions against a resistance for an extended period of time, e.g. the ability to perform 500 press-ups without rest.

Strength

Strength relates to your body's capacity to exert force on physical objects using muscles. Weightlifting is a good example of strength training as the aim is to condition the muscle to maximize its power, and often its size. Strength often comes at the expense of peak aerobic performance because muscle bulk prevents the body from moving efficiently.

Speed

Speed can relate to either the time taken to transport the whole body over a distance, or to co-ordinate joint actions. The development of speed is highly specific to the activity undertaken, e.g. sprinting or boxing. It depends on the level of flexibility and must be developed in parallel with strength. Speed is effectively a skill which must be pre-learned, rehearsed and perfected before it is done at high levels. Speed training is performed by using high-velocity movements for brief intervals in order to develop the correct neuromuscular pathways and energy sources used for the specific activity.

Flexibility

Flexibility refers to the ability of your joints to move through a full range of motions. Having flexibility in your muscles allows for more movement around the joints which improves endurance, strength and speed as well as making your body less susceptible to injury. Flexibility is developed through stretching exercises.

HOW IS FITNESS DEVELOPED?

Before you embark on a fitness regime you must first focus on what you want to achieve; what are you training to be 'fit' enough for? Whatever you decide on as your fitness goal, there are four basic principles that are the building blocks of every fitness programme, and which ultimately will determine how quickly and successfully you will achieve your training targets. These training principles are:

Frequency

How often you train. While as a general rule the more you train the quicker you will improve, it is possible to over-train, which can limit your progress.

Intensity

How hard you train. The aim is to progressively overload your body using incremental steps.

Time

How long you train for. This should be based on the type of activity you are engaged in and your training goal. For people returning to exercise or working towards a new goal, the time spent exercising should be increased as personal fitness develops.

Type

The type of exercise undertaken. According to training principles, the type of exercise conducted is derived from the aim of the exercise session or programme. Exercise

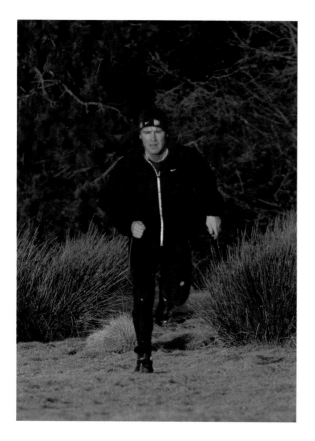

activities come in two main forms: aerobic (with oxygen) and anaerobic (without oxygen). The aim of aerobic exercise is to raise your heart rate into a training range for a sustained period (perhaps 30 minutes) and, therefore, cause your heart and lungs to work harder pumping oxygen to the muscles being used. In contrast, anaerobic exercise is short-burst exercise which is fuelled by the oxygen already in the muscles. The type and pace of anaerobic exercises prevents the body from replenishing the muscles with the oxygen they need to sustain the activity over a long period. Sprinting and weightlifting are two examples of anaerobic exercise. Exercises are rarely either aerobic or anaerobic, instead they sit somewhere on a scale between the two. On the battlefield, paratroopers must perform both aerobic and anaerobic activities, but the primary requirements are muscular and aerobic endurance and these requirements drive the type of fitness we undertake in training.

BUILDING A FITNESS PROGRAMME?

A fitness programme works by gradually getting your body to adapt to the demands placed on it during training. The most successful programmes target the specific gains that want to be achieved. For a training programme to be effective it must progressively overload the body in order for training outputs to continue to improve. The body can be overloaded by increasing the frequency, intensity or duration of exercise activity. However, to avoid injury and achieve maximum gains it is important that progression is gradual and only one overload principle (e.g. intensity) is increased per session. Above all else, it is important to keep up with the programme as all gains achieved by training are reversible; muscles deteriorate (atrophy), endurance is lost in a third of the time it takes to acquire, and strength also declines, albeit at a slower rate.

Variety is another key ingredient in every successful training programme as it combats boredom and reduces the risk of injury. As a general rule:

- Easy sessions should follow hard sessions.
- Rest should follow hard sessions.
- Long workouts should follow short workouts.
- Relaxed sessions should follow intense sessions.
- If training becomes boring, review the programme.

As I explained earlier, paratroopers need a balance between strength and cardiovascular fitness, which is what our training programme is designed to achieve and is ultimately what we test for during P Company. When training potential PARAS, we gradually increase the frequency, intensity and time of training sessions and every session has a goal. This goal alone dictates the type of training conducted. Paratroopers don't believe in 'junk sessions' put in to fill a programme, and neither should you. We need to have a goal and we need to get value from every session. Remember this and ask yourself what your goal is next time you train.

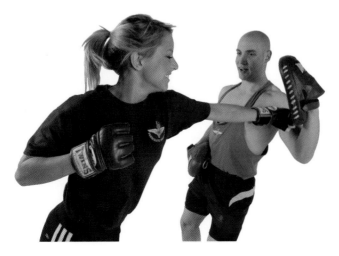

GAUGING TRAINING INTENSITY

Throughout the training programmes, you will see that much care has been taken to specify the intensity required for either the session or the activity. Below is a table which gives you two methods of judging your effort as a percentage of your exercise maximum.

TRAINING ZONE	SPARTAN METHOD	EMPEROR METHOD
Moderate activity zone: 50–60% effort	You are able to talk	50–60% of maximum heart rate
Weight management zone: 60–70% effort	You can use short sentences only	60–70% of maximum heart rate
Aerobic zone: 70–80% effort	You can utter a few words at a time	70–80% of maximum heart rate
Anaerobic threshold zone: 80–90% effort	You are only able to say one word at a time	80–90% of maximum heart rate
Redline zone: 90–100% effort	There is no chance of being able to talk	90–100% of maximum heart rate

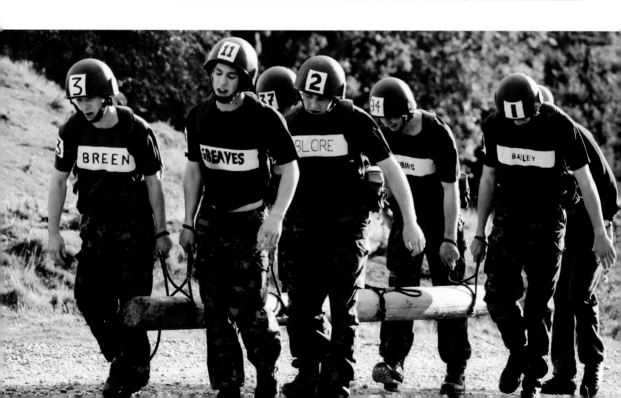

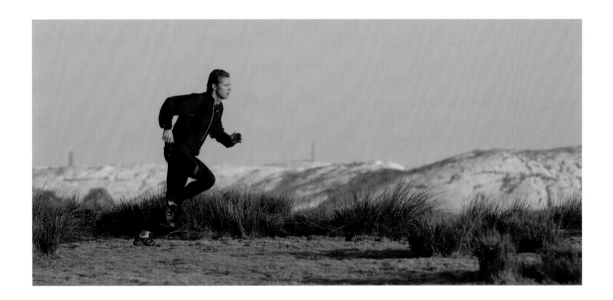

- **Moderate activity zone:** This training zone, while a pretty boring place to be, burns more fat than carbohydrates.
- **Weight management zone:** This zone strengthens your heart, giving it the opportunity to work at its optimum level for a sustained period.
- **Aerobic zone:** The aerobic zone benefits your heart and respiratory system and with it increases your endurance and aerobic power. In this zone you burn a higher proportion of carbohydrates than fats. It is the optimum zone to get fitter, faster and stronger.
- **Anaerobic threshold zone:** This training zone gives a training intensity where your body is just able to provide enough oxygen to power your muscles. The benefit is that it gradually increases the efficiency of your muscles at removing the exercise waste products such as lactic acid, thereby increasing your anaerobic threshold.
- **Redline zone:** This is the highest intensity training zone, which should not to be entered unless you are extremely fit. The redline zone is past the anaerobic threshold which means your muscles are using more oxygen than your body can provide.

To use your heart rate as a measure of training intensity you'll need to calculate your training zone as illustrated below and monitor it during training with a heart rate monitor.

TRAINING ZONE	START OF RANGE	END OF RANGE
50–60%	(.5 x 120) + 70 = 130	(.6 x 120) + 70 = 142
60–70%	(.6 x 120) + 70 = 142	(.7 x 120) + 70 = 154
70–80%	(.7 x 120) + 70 = 154	(.8 x 120) + 70 = 166
80–90%	(.8 x 120) + 70 = 166	(.9 x 120) + 70 = 178
90–100%	(.9 x 120) + 70 = 178	(1 x 120) + 70 = 190

CALCULATING YOUR TRAINING ZONES BY HEART RATE

- **Maximum:** The only true way to determine you maximum heart rate is to conduct a VO2 Max test; a highly technical assessment where the person being tested is taken to the extremes of their physical capacity, while having both their breathing and heart rate monitored. However, it can be approximated by taking your age away from 220. For a 30 year old, their maximum heart rate would be calculated as follows: 220 minus 30 = 190.
- **Resting heart rate:** Measure your heart rate for a minute in bed, just after you wake, e.g. 70.
- **Training range:** This can be calculated by subtracting your resting heart rate from your maximum heart rate, e.g. 190 minus 70 = 120.
- **Training zones:** To work out your training zones multiply your training range by the zone parameters as a decimal and add it to your resting heart rate.

Fighting Injury

At P Company we always work on the principle that prevention is better than cure, but unfortunately with any vigorous exercise programme injuries are inevitable. I have sustained many exercise-related injuries, including breaking my ankle twice, being reduced to walking with crutches through muscle and ligament damage, suffering heat exhaustion, and the initial stages of hypothermia. Nearly all of these could have been avoided. You can prevent most injuries by respecting your body and respecting your exercise environment by identifying potential hazards and then avoiding them. Beyond that it is important that you make sure you are doing the exercises correctly and that you take time to warm up and cool down properly for each session.

The human body has evolved into an incredibly advanced biological system and pain is its way of signalling that something is wrong. The more you exercise, the more you'll be able to identify whether any pain is serious, but in general terms, if you suffer anything more than minor discomfort you should stop exercising.
If in any doubt consult your doctor.

TRAINING THROUGH INJURIES

Sustaining an injury during an exercise programme can be a real blow, but training through it will only compound and prolong the effects of the injury. For example, if you continue running on a sprained ankle, it will almost certainly affect your biomechanics and change your gait. In my experience the use of drugs to deal with an injury can be extremely dangerous. While anti-inflammatory drugs and painkillers can help in the short term, they typically deal with the effect rather than the cause of the injury. Masking the pain and forcing your body to run in an unnatural way increases the risk of secondary injuries, which can potentially be even more serious than the initial injury. During my time at P Company an RAF officer boldly attempted the 20-mile endurance march with stress fractures in his shins, which we didn't know at the time. The result of 20 miles of pounding with an unnatural gait was a broken pelvis – an injury which has the potential to paralyze or even be life-threatening due to its proximity to a major artery. With an injury it is possible to win the battle, but lose the war. In my opinion, it is never worth putting at risk your chance of reaching your goal for the sake of a couple of training sessions. Listen to your body and rest. In most cases you will be able to reschedule your training, or do an alternative exercise. For instance, if you sprain your ankle replace your run with a swim, which will not only deliver the same training value in a similar time, but will aid your recovery by keeping your ankle mobile without the threat of worsening the injury.

HOW TO PREVENT AND CURE SOME COMMON INJURIES

DEHYDRATION

Dehydration is a potentially fatal condition. It's well known that nearly two-thirds of all your body's cells are made up of water. During exercise your muscles generate heat, which your body regulates through sweating in order to prevent you from cooking alive. Your level of fitness, combined with your clothing and your exercise environment, will determine how efficiently your body controls heat generated by exercise. Above all, however, water is your greatest ally in fighting off dehydration. The chart below identifies the associated symptoms and risks with varying degrees of dehydration.

Dehydration	Symptoms
1%	Feeling thirsty.
2%	Loss of appetite and a 20% reduction in physical performance.

4%	Tiredness, nausea and a feeling of drunkenness.
6%	Irritability and aggressiveness.
10%	The body loses the ability to regulate its temperature.
11%	The body starts to break down proteins responsible for bodily function, making simple muscle movement close to impossible.
21%	Death.

The Immediate Action Drill for an injury caused by trauma is *PRICE*:

- Protect
- Rest
- Ice
- Compression
- Elevation

As shown above it is vital that you drink sufficient water before, during and after exercise to ensure you are hydrated; even marginal dehydration can seriously inhibit your performance and, therefore, the value you get from your session. Plan on consuming 500ml of water per hour spent exercising and if your urine isn't clear, drink some more – you are already dehydrated!

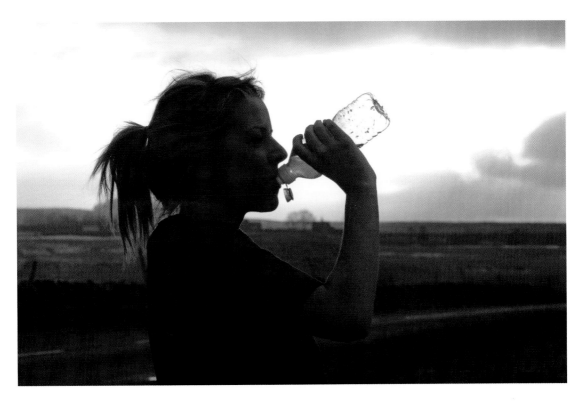

SPRAINED ANKLE

Cause: An over-stretching or tearing of supporting ligaments.

Symptoms: Local inflammation, pain and bruising.

Prevention: Careful footing over uneven terrain. Improve ligament strength using leg balancing exercises. Try standing on one leg and throwing a ball against a wall using alternate hands.

ILIOTIBIAL BAND (ITB) SYNDROME

Cause: Lazy gluteal muscles and poor pre- and post-exercise stretch discipline.

Symptoms: Acute pain in the vicinity of the knee cap while running.

Prevention: Comprehensive warm-up and cool-down before and after exercise and glute strengthening exercises. If suffered, try rowing with a resistance band tied just above your knee.

ACHILLES TENDONITIS

Cause: Over-training, badly fitting (rubbing) shoes and poor stretching regime.

Symptoms: Inflammation and tenderness at the back of the heel.

Prevention: Calf stretching before and after exercise, ensuring sufficient rest in-between sessions and wearing the right footwear. If sustained, spend as much time as you can stretching and massaging the area and avoid activities which aggravate the symptoms.

SHIN SPLINTS

Cause: Over-training, following a programme with too much impact or not changing running shoes frequently enough.

Symptoms: A dull ache felt along the front of the shin bone.

Prevention: Alternating between high- and low-impact training sessions during your training programme and changing running shoes regularly. If developed, use alternative exercises until the symptoms disappear.

MUSCLE TEARS

Cause: Over-training, hyperextension from a sudden movement, or too many repetitions of the same exercise.

Symptoms: Feeling a sudden, painful tearing sensation which turns into an acute pain in the muscle.

Prevention: Thorough warm-up and stretching before working out and taking care to gradually increase the frequency and intensity of sessions. If suffered, rest and engage in activities that exercise different parts of the body.

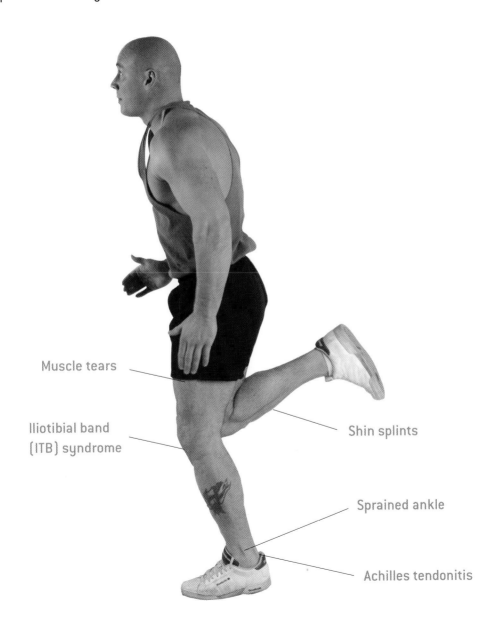

Muscle tears

Iliotibial band (ITB) syndrome

Shin splints

Sprained ankle

Achilles tendonitis

Food is Fuel

You don't run a Ferrari on diesel and nor will a paratrooper perform if he is fed on junk food. The food you eat not only affects your energy for exercise but your general health and well-being. It is important to maintain a healthy, balanced diet containing a variety of foods including: plenty of fruit and vegetables; plenty of starchy foods such as wholegrain bread, pasta and rice; some protein-rich foods such as meat, fish, eggs and lentils; and some dairy foods. It should also be low in fat (especially saturated fat), salt and sugar.

ENERGY AND STORAGE

Think of your body as a calorie bank account. If you consume more calories than you use your energy balance increases, and vice versa. The body stores excess energy as fat, to be burned at a later date. Every 3,500 calories equates to 1lb of fat. Therefore, to lose weight your calorie intake must be less than your calorie expenditure. The fewer calories you eat and the more you exercise regularly, the more fat you will burn. However, while intensive workouts like high-impact aerobics or rowing burn more calories than lightweight training, gaining muscle mass is crucial to weight loss. Muscles require calories just to keep them at their current size. Therefore the more muscle mass you have the more calories you burn, even when you are resting.

CALORIE-BURNING CALCULATOR				
Rank	Activity (1 hour)	Calories burnt (per lb per minute)	Calories burnt per hour by 12-stone (168lb) person Weight (lb) x time (min) x calories burnt (cal/lb/min)	Time taken to burn 1lb of fat
1	Bicycling: >20mph Running: 10mph (6-min mile)	0.1211	e.g. 168 x 60 x .1211 = 1220	2hrs 52min
2	Boxing: in ring Rowing: vigorous effort Rock climbing: ascending rock	0.0908	915	3hrs 49min
3	Rugby Running: 6mph (10-min mile) Football: competitive Swimming laps: freestyle, vigorous effort	0.0757	763	4hrs 35min
4	Rowing: moderate effort Circuit training Rock climbing: descending Swimming laps: freestyle, moderate effort	0.0605	610	5hrs 24min
5	Aerobics: high-impact Soccer: recreational Tennis: recreational	0.0530	534	6hrs 33min
6	Aerobics: moderate effort Boxing: punching bag Dancing: aerobic (ballet or salsa) Bicycling: 10mph, leisure	0.0454	457	7hrs 39min
7	Golf Dancing: moderate	0.0416	419	8hrs 20min
8	Walking: 4mph, very brisk pace	0.0302	305	11hrs 30min
9	Walking: 3mph, moderate pace, e.g. walking a dog	0.0265	267	13hrs 7min
10	Watching TV	0.0090	91	38hrs 26min

EATING FOR EXERCISE

Exercise uses up energy and fluids. To get the most out of your exercise programme you should:

- Drink plenty of fluids.
- Consume plenty of wholegrain breads and cereals, fruit and vegetables and moderate amounts of milk, yoghurt and cheese, lean meat, fish, poultry, eggs, nuts and pulses.
- Maintain energy levels during exercise with carbohydrates.
- Tailor your meal portions to your level of exercise activity.
- Avoiding eating a large meal within two hours of commencing exercise.
- Eat as soon as possible after exercise; for the first two hours after exercise, muscles can refuel their glycogen stores (from carbohydrate-containing foods) twice as fast as normal.

CARB-UP FOR ENERGY

Eating carbohydrates fuels the glycogen stores in your muscles, which determine how long you can perform; this is particularly important in endurance activities. Foods rich in starchy carbohydrates, such as bread, rice, pasta, cereals and potatoes, are best followed closely by fruit, vegetables, beans, pulses, yoghurt and milk.

PROTEIN FOR REPAIR AND BULK

Protein's primary dietary function is to maintain muscle growth and repair. While it is a secondary source of energy, it won't improve aerobic performance. Very active people, who train frequently, generally require more protein than those who don't. However, contrary to popular belief, most people in the Western world eat more protein than they need, so even the very active should get enough protein from their diet.

SPORT SUPPLEMENTS

While sports supplements provide a precise and convenient method of taking specific nutrients, you should be able to get all the nutrients you need from a healthy, balanced diet and supplements won't make up for eating poorly. If you take supplements, pay careful attention to their calorific content or you may end up storing the energy as fat not muscle.

Kit & Equipment

I have heard some people say that a good workman never blames his tools, but find me a good workman who uses bad ones. In the PARAS we pride ourselves on looking after our kit, as on operations even the simplest items have the ability to transform, or even save, your life. During P Company we instil in recruits the importance of ensuring that their kit is fit for purpose and of looking after it. The wrong, or badly fitting, kit makes even the most moderate of tasks impossible. Having experienced the effects of badly fitting boots and a poorly packed Bergen, these are not mistakes I will repeat. In a physical training environment the wrong kit can cause injuries that unhinge your entire training programme. The following list is by no means exhaustive, but it will give you an idea of what is important and what you can do without.

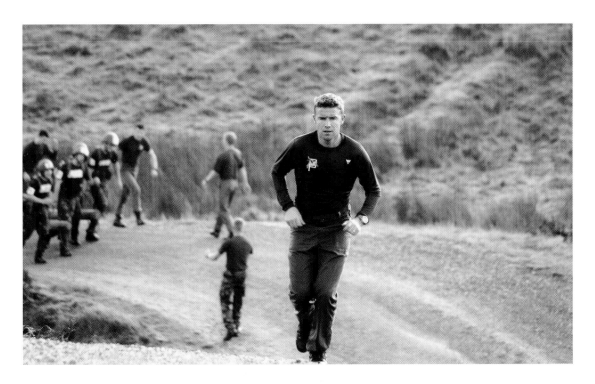

THE ESSENTIALS

TRAINING SHOES

Your training shoes are perhaps the most important element of your fitness kit and, therefore, it is worth investing time and money to make sure you get the right ones for you. As a general rule it is best to go to a specialist sports shop to be fitted for a shoe that meets all your requirements. However, if you're not able to do this, here are some tips.

Size matters

Your feet swell during exercise, so consider getting shoes half a size larger than your normal ones. Also, take particular care in ensuring that the shoe is wide enough as well as long enough.

Cushioning

When you run, your training shoe has to absorb three times your body weight. If you are a heavy runner, or have a history of compression injuries, find a training shoe with extra cushioning.

Fit for the task

You need to select a training shoe which is appropriate for the surface you will mostly be running on. Whether you are road running, off-road running or a combination of the two, find a shoe which is designed for the purpose. If in doubt, find a hybrid trainer, which will have a tread deep enough to cope with running both on and off road.

Specialist running shoes

Runners typically run in one of three ways in terms of how they land: overpronation (flat-footed), neutral (normal) or underpronation (high-arched feet). This affects the sort of shoe that is most suitable for the individual. Different training shoes are designed to offer appropriate support for each type of running. If in

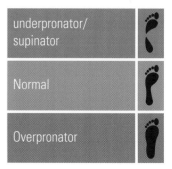

underpronator/ supinator

Normal

Overpronator

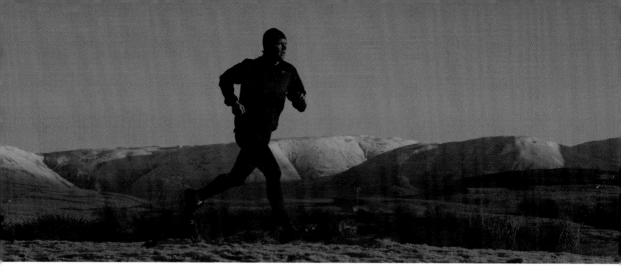

doubt, go to a shop that offers specialist fitting. Alternatively, examine the print left by your foot after a bath or shower to see how you land.

Replacing your shoes

As you would expect, the more you run, the more often you will need to change your shoes. As a rule you should aim to change your trainers every 500–600 miles.

How much?

This depends entirely on your ego. While your knees will absorb the cost of a cheap pair of trainers, the most expensive pair won't necessarily be the best. I'd recommend getting last year's model and using the internet to source the best price.

CLOTHING

Good clothes won't turn a shire horse into a thoroughbred, but they will make you feel more comfortable and, therefore, more likely to train.

Shorts

Whatever your preferred style, find shorts that are made of a lightweight and breathable material. Select a size and style that will reduce chafing between your legs. However, if you do suffer from this, Vaseline is another good solution.

Tops

Like your shorts, you are looking for a top which is lightweight, breathable and made of a material that will wick the sweat away from your body. Once you have taken those criteria into consideration, the style you choose is really a combination of personal preference and finding something appropriate for your training environment.

Leggings

I think running leggings are brilliant. They are much lighter than tracksuit bottoms, but keep you just as warm. If you often run in winter, and can pull it off, get a pair.

Jackets

Running in winter can be made much more bearable with the right jacket. Look for a breathable, waterproof jacket which will not only keep you dry, but also provide a barrier against the wind.

Socks

While I am prone to going without socks, they do provide a barrier that protects your feet against rubbing and your shoes from stinking. It is possible to spend a lot on a pair of technical socks that offers anti-blister protection, extra cushioning or aids circulation, but I think it is better to find a pair that is comfortable and within your price range.

Watch

You need a watch to keep track of how long you are training for. You don't need anything fancy and a good starting point is a waterproof watch with a stopwatch, lap counter and countdown facility.

LUXURIES

There is a vast array of equipment cleverly designed to aid your training and separate you from your hard-earned cash. However, here are a few that can make a real difference.

MUSIC IS THE ANSWER

Disassociation is when something takes your mind off training so much that it enables you to maintain the same performance while making you more relaxed and lowering your heart rate. In this domain the MP3 player is king.

Find the right music and your trip to the dojo will feel more like a trip to the disco. Like most electrical items, MP3 players are getting much cheaper. Look for one that is light and small enough to clip on your shorts without affecting them. Next, make sure your earphones will stay in your ears with all the jolts and sweat caused by exercise.

LISTEN TO YOUR HEART

Using a heart rate monitor is great way to capture your body's reaction to exercise, and identifying specific performance levels. It is also possible to use one to identify when you are suffering from an infection and resting would be better. They are becoming increasing affordable, but the more advanced models still command a high price. Heart rate monitors offer a broad spectrum of functions including:

- Current, maximum, minimum and average heart rate.
- Audio alerts covering specific training zones.
- Capability to upload training record to PC.
- GPS and altimeter.

TRACKING YOUR TRAINING

While GPS (Global Positioning System) devices have been around for years, up until fairly recently you wouldn't have wanted to take one running with you unless it was to defend yourself against an attacker. But as I keep saying, results are the ultimate motivator, and the GPS enables you to track your progress perfectly. The appeal of a GPS is not knowing your precise location to within 5m, but instead knowing exactly how long, fast and high you've been running; by uploading the information onto your PC. While watch variants are expensive, relatively bulky and thirsty for battery power, it is possible to find a GPS for a relatively modest price.

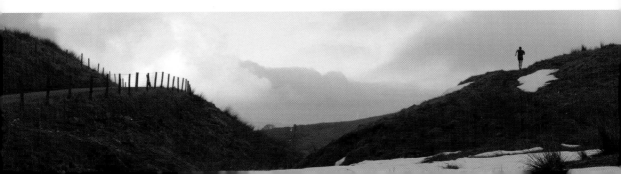

THE BRUNEVAL RAID – OPERATION *BITING*
Overcoming fear and anxiety through goal setting

In 1942, RAF bombers were incurring heavy losses. These were caused by advances in German radar technology, which was increasingly able to locate RAF aircraft at a distance. They would then be intercepted by German fighters and destroyed before they could carry out their mission. British scientists were eager to understand German advances in order to create countermeasures to neutralize their effect and advance the Allies' own radars. A German radar located on the coast at Bruneval, in northern France, was identified as a suitable site to capture both radar and operators for interrogation. However, it was concluded that an amphibious operation was likely to incur heavy casualties due to the proximity of local reinforcements and naval patrol boats. Therefore, the only solution was an airborne raid.

Operation *Biting* fell to C Company, 2 PARA, commanded by Major John Frost. Major Frost's plan was for a night-time airborne insertion of 130 men, who would then be extracted after the raid by naval landing craft. However, the PARAS faced several significant challenges before they even left England. C Company had only just been formed and fewer than half its men were parachute-trained, with even fewer being able to swim – which was necessary for them to reach the landing craft. Parachuting was in its infancy and none of the RAF pilots assigned to the mission had conducted a drop. Information on the radar station was scant and little was known about the German guard strength or the speed and strength of local German Army reserves. This would be the first operational descent for the PARAS, and not only would the safety of the RAF bombers depend on the mission being a success, but so too would the future of the Parachute Regiment.

C Company commenced a consolidated period of training and rehearsal for the raid, continually improving their plan with the RAF and Royal Navy units supporting them. Major Frost's first challenge

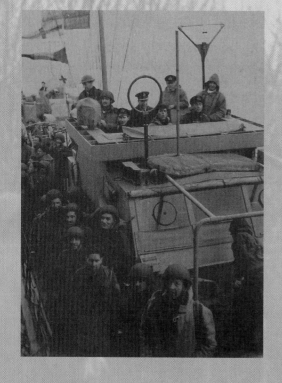

A motor gun boat brings Major Frost and the men of 2 PARA home in triumph after the raid.

was to ensure that no soldier was fazed by either the insertion or the extraction, so mastering swimming and parachuting was their first goal. Secondly, the company built a scale model of the radar station on the bank of a Scottish loch and practised each aspect of the plan separately: the insertion, the attack, the dismantling of the radar equipment, the extraction of the equipment and radar operators to the boat RV and the extraction by landing craft. Finally, C Company put all of the parts of the plan together and drilled it until everyone knew their part perfectly. In parallel the Royal Navy and RAF analyzed the environmental factors that would best ensure success – identifying that a raid in late February would give C Company the perfect combination of clear skies, high tide and a long period of darkness to conduct their mission.

On the evening of 27 February 1942, Operation *Biting* was launched and was a complete success. C Company suffered only a few casualties during the raid and captured both radar equipment and operators, which ultimately proved the capability of airborne forces and led to the RAF developing effective counter-measures for German radars, saving a countless number of lives.

The Bruneval raid is still widely acknowledged as a brilliantly executed airborne operation and I believe there are many lessons that can be transferred into any highly stressed performance setting. By analyzing the mission, Major Frost was able to break the task down into proximate goals (learning to swim, breaking down

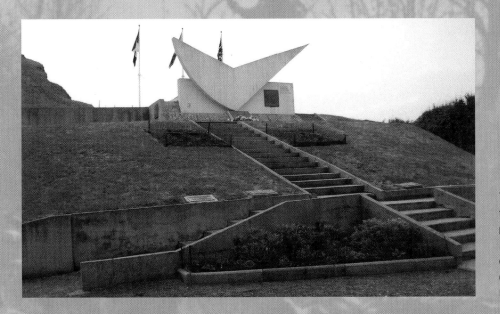

This monument to the men who took part in Operation *Biting* is on the site of the German defences at Bruneval.

A battle map of the Bruneval raid showing the major objectives and strong German defences.

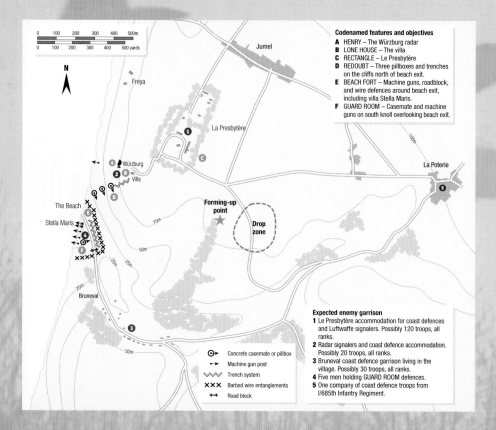

Codenamed features and objectives
A HENRY – The Würzburg radar
B LONE HOUSE – The villa
C RECTANGLE – Le Presbytère
D REDOUBT – Three pillboxes and trenches on the cliffs north of beach exit.
E BEACH FORT – Machine guns, roadblock, and wire defences around beach exit, including villa Stella Maris.
F GUARD ROOM – Casemate and machine guns on south knoll overlooking beach exit.

Expected enemy garrison
1 Le Presbytère accommodation for coast defences and Luftwaffe signalers. Possibly 120 troops, all ranks.
2 Radar signalers and coast defence accommodation. Possibly 20 troops, all ranks.
3 Bruneval coast defence garrison living in the village. Possibly 30 troops, all ranks.
4 Five men holding GUARD ROOM defences.
5 One company of coast defence troops from I/685th Infantry Regiment.

Concrete casemate or pillbox
Machine gun post
Trench system
Barbed wire entanglements
Road block

a radar, etc). This prevented C Company from being overwhelmed by the enormity of their task, as they only switched to the whole task when they had mastered the component parts. By isolating the company for training, Frost was able to remove any external pressure and focus everyone on the task at hand rather than on the consequences of failure. By integrating the RAF and Royal Navy into his planning, he was able to use their expertise to conduct specific PARA and amphibious training, as well as to identify the ideal timing for the raid – leaving C Company to focus on getting the ground plan right.

Regardless of the challenges you choose to undertake I would recommend using the following three steps to help you overcome your performance anxiety:

- Break the challenge down into its component parts and only put these together when you have mastered them individually.
- Create the most realistic setting to rehearse your plan.
- Use the expertise of those around you to refine your plan of attack as much as is possible.

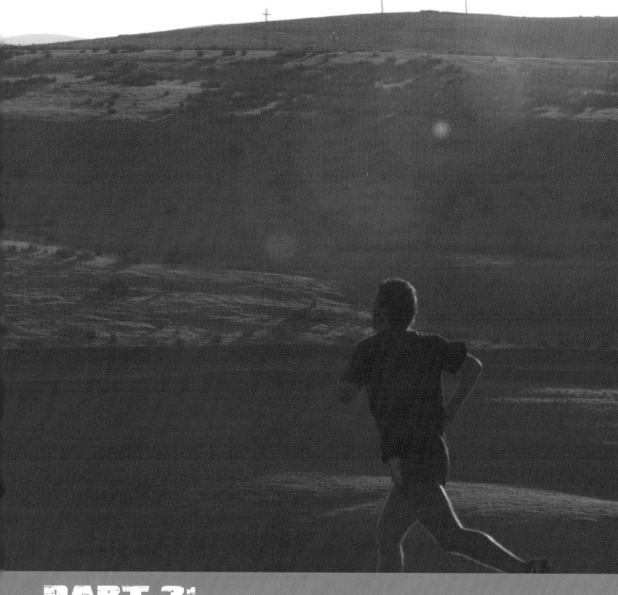

PART 3:
PREPARING FOR WAR

'Strategy without tactics is the slowest route to victory. Tactics without strategy is the noise before defeat.'

Sun Tzu

On operational tour in the
Western Desert, Iraq, 2006.

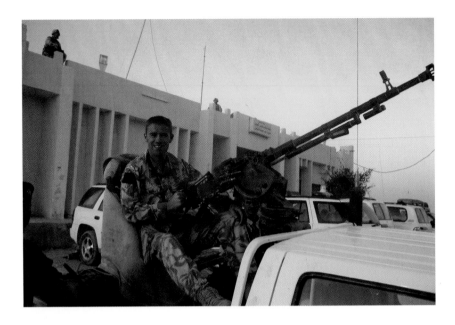

We have discussed physical preparation and now we will go on to look at mental preparation – not only how you plan the mission, but how you think of the mission.

As a Parachute Regiment commander, I have been involved in the planning and execution of many combat missions. One of my commanding officers once told me that second-place trophies in our business mean death and destruction, which certainly focuses the mind. Besides the quality of the people I have had the pleasure of working with, it has been our collective approach that has kept us winning the gold medal.

Before we do anything, we first focus on the aim of our mission. This must be clear, and the prize for success must always at least be worth the cost of success and the possible consequences of failure. In the example of the Bruneval raid, the goal was to capture the enemy radar, a goal that was both clear and had demonstrable value to the war effort. However, within the goal there were a number of subordinate goals integral to its success; completing a PARA insertion, defeating the Germans, capturing and extracting the radar and its operators, securing the beachhead, meeting the boats and then extracting the equipment and operators for interrogation. Together, all of these goals were equally important. For each, painstaking thought and planning went into guaranteeing their success.

In particular, by analyzing the factors of ground, enemy, time, space and resources, 2 PARA were able to create and rehearse a plan for each goal in order to create the highest chance of success.

While much of the technology of warfare has changed in the past 65 years, in essence our approach to executing missions is exactly the same as that used by 2 PARA at Bruneval. Once we have devised a workable plan, we refine it through a process of war gaming. The war game is used to:

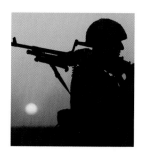

- Deconflict tasks and resources in time and space.
- Identify potential strengths in the plan and exploit them.
- Identify potential weaknesses in the plan and find solutions for them.

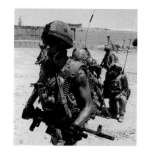

The war game relies on harnessing the expertise of every member involved in the plan to make success on the battlefield as swift and certain as possible. At the end of our war games we always end up with a better plan, but perhaps even more useful is the shared experience of anticipating, talking and thinking through the potential interactions between us and the enemy. Success on the battlefield is based on the commitment and understanding of everyone involved. We will deal with commitment first.

As I mentioned earlier, in my experience paratroopers only commit to a plan when they instinctively feel it is worthwhile and will succeed. However, a brilliant plan is never enough. It must also be communicated well to those integral to making it succeed. In my opinion, a full rehearsal is a battle winner, but often time and space conspire to make that impossible. In these instances, we always use a model detailing all the key features of a plan so that we can run through all aspects of it in chronological order, detailing each person's role and activity. Time is spent talking through what will happen in certain circumstances. Where issues are identified, they are discussed and resolved. The result of these discussions, if well run, is that all involved have an excellent level of comprehension of the plan.

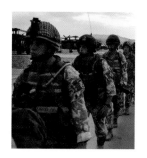

In this chapter, I will explain how to adapt the PARA approach to mission planning to your new exercise regime.

Change – The Aim of your Programm

In the PARAS one of our main battle planning principles is that you never reinforce failure, for to do so wastes lives and resources. If something isn't working you need to change your approach. After all, if you keep doing what you've always done, you'll get the same results you've always got. All major advances in science, technology, business and relationships result from a fundamental change – your health is no different! A new fitness regime equates to a significant change in your diet and exercise habits and this is why you need to be on a war footing.

Drawing on much research into change, I have concluded that effective change follows three steps:

- **Unfreezing:** Identifying that change is required.
- **Changing:** Continually evaluating new approaches that move you towards to your desired state.
- **Refreezing:** Adopting your new approaches.

Other research into personal change has proved that the secret to success is doing a new activity 21 times in close succession for it to be adopted as a habit. As stated in the introduction, stick to this programme for five weeks and your approach to fitness will change forever.

GOAL-SETTING

In the same way that PARAS need a specific mission to focus their efforts on, so too do you. Your fitness mission, or goal, is the basis of everything you do in your programme and, like the Bruneval raid, it will be made up of many subordinate goals. Goal-setting is now common practice in business, sport and education, but research has shown that for it to work you need to believe that your performance goal is something attainable, rather than an ability that others are born with. When setting your goal it should follow SMART criteria as illustrated in the examples below.

	Health goal	Performance goal
Specific	Lose weight	Run a marathon
Measureable	Two stone	In under four hours
Achievable Do you have sufficient time, knowledge, skills and physical resources to achieve this?	Yes	Yes
Relevant Is this relevant to your wider goal?	Yes	Yes
Time-specific	By 15 March	On 26 April

Research into goal-setting proved that:

- Goals must be challenging, but achievable: if they are too easy, the goal will be perceived as boring and unlikely to instigate action; if they are too difficult, the goal will be demotivating.
- Feedback enhances the effectiveness of goal-setting, enabling you to adjust your behaviour in order to achieve your goal.
- Specific goals (e.g. running this year's London marathon in under three hours) are more effective than general goals (e.g. getting fitter), because they provide objective criteria to measure your performance against.
- Proximal (short-term) goals have more motivational impact than distal (long-term) goals, because they provide quicker feedback on progress.

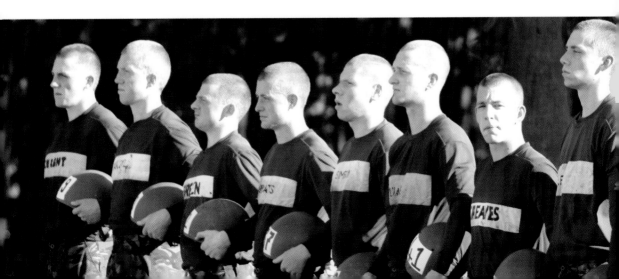

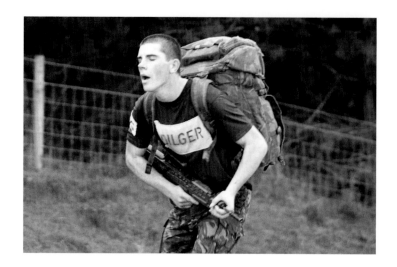

Once you have identified your performance goal, the next challenge is to maintain your motivation for achieving it. This motivation will be determined by the following: external factors (e.g. positive feedback); interactive factors (e.g. a public goal such as fear of public failure) and internal factors (e.g. self-efficacy). As internal factors are the ones you have the most control over I will explain how self-efficacy works in a bit more detail.

SELF-EFFICACY

Self-efficacy is your perception of your ability to achieve your goal. This belief must have two components: first, that specific activities will deliver specific results (e.g. circuit training three times a week burns fat and builds muscle), and second that you believe in your own ability (e.g. you are able to take part in circuit training). Self-belief is typically based on the following four factors:

- Previous relevant (to goal) performance.
- Modelling – comparing yourself to a known person who has accomplished a similar performance goal.
- Being told you're capable of the performance goal by someone whom you believe to have relevant knowledge or experience.
- Your state of mind – how happy, sad or anxious you are at a given time.

In order to get the best from goal-setting, it is important to constantly evaluate your goal so you can adapt it to changes that are outside your control (e.g. a race being cancelled). Also, always go for goal quality over goal quantity.

Mission Planning

I now need you to get your head into a war setting. Significantly improving your fitness equates to sustained lifestyle change; your plan to achieve it needs to be flawless and you need to secure the support and commitment of your family, friends and colleagues to make it work. I need you to complete the planning process on pages 190–191, using the one on pages 72–73 as an example. Your objective is to find sufficient space for the number and duration of the workouts you want to include per week – your target is four sessions.

Now having spent time planning where you'll find time to exercise, look through your weekly timeline again and identify the weaknesses in your plan. If you struggle getting up in the morning, this might not be the best time to exercise. Is it possible to run or cycle to work? Could you eat lunch at your desk and squeeze a session in during your lunch break? If you go for a drink with your friends after work every day, replacing even one of these will deliver a double benefit: calories are burned training and not consumed drinking. You also need to give thought to your eating habits – you need at least 1–2 hours after eating before exercising and you need to be sober. I believe that exercise should never be taken at the expense of your family commitments, but maybe there is a compromise – one of my friends runs with his dog and his daughters cycling alongside three times a week; he gets quality time with his kids and a workout all in one. Is there anything else in your timeline that you think would benefit from being changed?

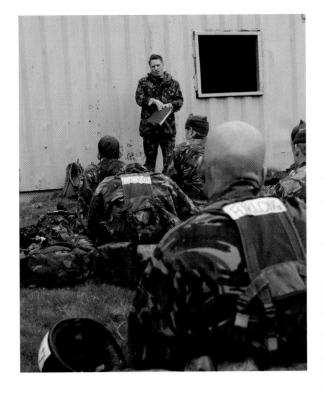

Now it's time to bring in the people who you think are key to the success of your fitness goal. In the PARAS this phase follows a comprehensive brief; which I wouldn't recommend in this instance, but I'd definitely advise you explaining to the key people you've identified the what, why and how of your plan, and in particular the help and support you need from them to make it possible.

The origins of your goal should form the 'why'. I'd leave the 'what' as simple as 'four one-hour fitness sessions' unless they have a particular interest in fitness. The 'how' is what you need to focus their attention on. I promise you, this process will not only show your key people that you're serious about your goals but it will make your method of achieving them significantly more robust.

Objective: Fill a time line of your typical week in order to identify:
1. Suitable windows for training – exploit.
2. Events which have the ability to cannibalize your fitness goal – avoid.

	Sleep	Work on maintaining at least seven hours. If anything you will need more when you are exercising.
	Work/College	Is there scope to train on your way to or from work/college or during your lunch break?
	Commitments	Any event which is important to you or your family and friends.
	Potential Pitfalls	These are events or potential events that could either stop you from training or eliminate the benefit you are getting from training.
	Opportunities	Free time to train.
	Fuel	Put your food in last, unless it is a social occasion. You should aim to plan your diet around your activities. For guidance see page 56.

FITNESS TRAINING BATTLE PLAN

	0100	0300	0500	0700	0900	1100
Monday						
Tuesday						
Wednesday						
Thursday						
Friday						
Saturday						
Sunday						

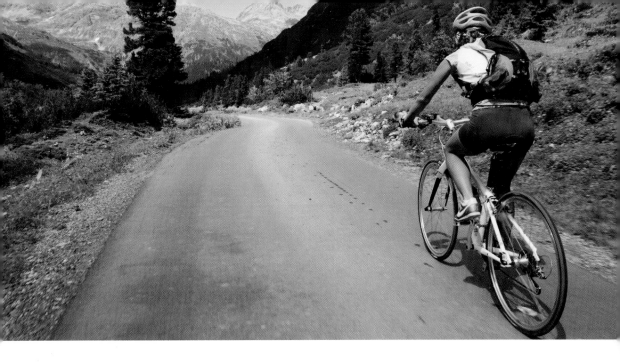

Critical Success Factors?

1. **Time:** How long do I need for each training session? (Include travel and changing time.)
2. **Resources:** What space and equipment do I need before or after my session? (Sports kit, spare work clothes, shower, food etc.)
3. **Fuel:** How do I need to manage the where, when and what I eat in order to be able to train?
4. **Win-Win:** How do I score a double victory, replacing a potential pitfall with a training session?
5. **Redundancy:** Where can I find additional sessions if I need to?
6. **Friendly Forces:** Whose help do I need to secure to be able to achieve my goal and how can I sell it to them?
7. **Enemies:** Who, where and what do I need to avoid in order to guarantee success?

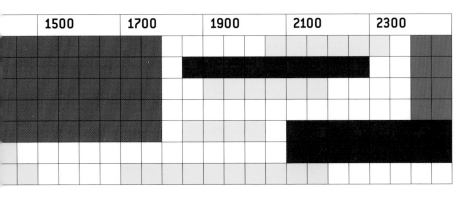

1500	1700	1900	2100	2300

Motivation

The issue of human motivation is so widely written about that you could fill a catalogue with books on the topic and still only scratch the surface. Motivation can be classified into two types: extrinsic and intrinsic motivation. Extrinsic motivation is when you do something to receive a reward or avoid a punishment. Intrinsic motivation is when you get pleasure or value from the activity itself. It has taken me a while, but I believe I am now intrinsically motivated to keep fit. Let me explain how.

Self-Determination Theory (SDT), perhaps the best known intrinsic motivation theory, seeks to explain how individuals aspire to grow to achieve their potential. The building blocks of SDT are that individuals will only achieve their potential if they achieve three psychological needs, which support intrinsic motivation: autonomy, relatedness and competence. Autonomy is the feeling that you are doing an activity through your own free will. Relatedness is the feeling that you like and are like others taking part in this activity. Competence relates to you viewing yourself as capable and competent in controlling the environment and being able to reliably predict outcomes.

SDT suggests that through time and experience it is possible for something to go from being extrinsically motivated to being intrinsically motivated. I will now use SDT to explain how I have become intrinsically motivated to exercise and, therefore, how you can too.

EXTERNAL REGULATION

Where a particular activity is influenced by the desire to attain a tangible reward, or avoid a threatened punishment; this is often demotivating.

> I started running three miles, five days a week, when I was 16 solely to get fit enough to join the PARAS. For me, the reward I sought was being accepted, whereas the punishment I was trying to avoid was failing the PARA entry standard.

INTROJECTION

Where a particular activity is influenced by the individual's perceived belief in the consequences, such as feelings of pride, guilt or shame, and thus the individual regulates their behaviour to either achieve or avoid these feelings. While introjections are internally regulated actions, they are not necessarily a self-determined behaviour and are, therefore, a relatively unstable form of regulation.

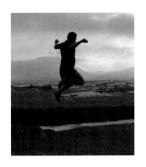

> During the two years I spent running five days a week before joining the PARAS, there were many things I'd rather have done in the morning. However, a combination of guilt and not wanting to fail the PARA entrance test kept me getting up at 0630hrs.

IDENTIFICATION

Where the individual identifies with the underlying value of an activity.

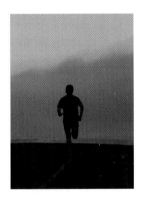

> After a couple of months I started to like the feeling I got from being fit and looking in better shape, which I knew was due to my running. At that point I wasn't experiencing enjoyment and satisfaction from the actual running, but that was exactly what my new-found physique and fitness was giving me.

INTEGRATION

Where an activity is performed for its own enjoyment and satisfaction. The most complete form of internalization of extrinsic motivation, which identifies the importance of an activity and is a source of fulfilment in itself.

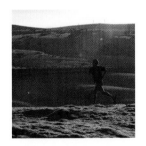

> When I took part in my first-ever Basic Fitness Test (the PARA 1½-mile run), I completed it in just over seven minutes, passing the test and winning the race by nearly a minute. This was the first race that I had ever won and it gave me an incredible feeling of achievement. Winning races wasn't an innate ability, it was something I acquired through running. That day I decided that I wanted to feel it again, and so I trained even harder. Gradually, I came to associate the feeling of winning with running, which not only made me want to do it more, but made me enjoy training for winning as well. Running became important to me and I've won every Basic Fitness Test since then.

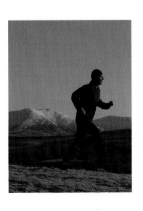

I believe this is exactly what you will experience when you achieve your goal. At first it feels as though you are only exercising for the goal, but quickly exercise will become a part of your lifestyle and you will feel guilty when you skip a session. Shortly after the guilt phase, you will start to feel and see the benefits of your exercise programme and you will enjoy them – they will be reason enough to keep you exercising. Then, when you achieve your goal, provided that attaining it has been hard enough to significantly challenge you, you will feel an incredible sense of achievement and you will want to taste that feeling of success again. You will keep exercising because you enjoy it and you will be hungry to build on your success and achieve some even more impressive goals.

MOTIVATIONAL EXERCISE

Human motivation is a uniquely personal emotion, but as a rule people tend to be extrinsically motivated to do something – motivated towards success or away from failure. The trick is to be able to identify what the positive and negative things are that will help you stay on track with

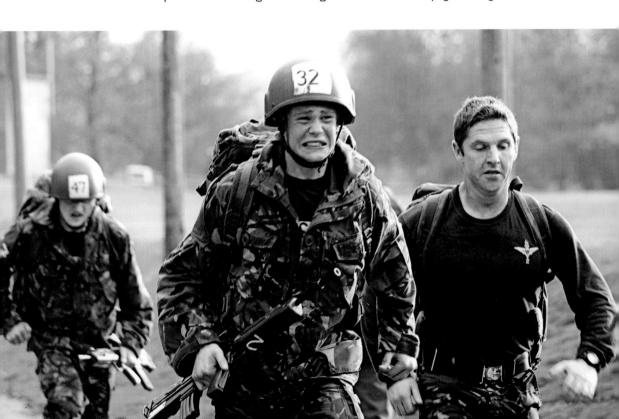

your new training programme. I believe the best method of identifying these factors is by evaluating the two different courses of action you have in terms of pain and pleasure. On a blank piece of paper, using the example below, write down the pain and pleasure you think you'll get from both starting a new fitness regime and doing nothing differently. As illustrated in the example, highlight specifically the pleasure you associate with getting fit (motivation towards success) and the pain you associate with doing nothing (motivation away from failure) – these are your carrots and sticks. What you now need to do is work out which motivation is more powerful for you and keep it at the forefront of your mind over the first five weeks of your training programme.

START YOUR NEW FITNESS REGIME		DO NOTHING	
Pain	Pleasure	Pain	Pleasure
Risk of injury	Feeling good	Loss of self-respect	Easy
Feeling embarrassed	Health benefits	Feeling embarrassed	Can continue with current lifestyle
Don't know how	Losing weight	Feeling lazy	
Feeling discomfort	Greater self-esteem	Less healthy	Getting progressively less healthy
Hard work	Gaining confidence	Risk to long-term health	
Less free time	Meeting new people		
	Relieving stress		

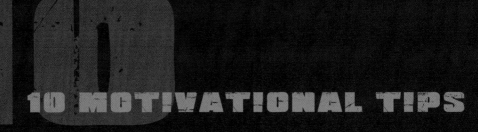

10 MOTIVATIONAL TIPS

1. **Results will keep you motivated**

   Continually refer to your goals and check your progress. Don't be afraid to review and change the plan if it's not working for you.

2. **Find a partner**

   You will be able to talk about your exercise experiences with someone who understands them completely and you won't want to let each other down.

3. **Do activities you like**

   The more you can do to make the programme feel like fun, the more likely you are to continue.

4. **Take an identical picture of yourself every four weeks**

   You will be able to see the effects your programme has on your appearance.

5. **Keep a training journal**

   Once every week take time to reflect on all you've achieved since you started out.

6. **Tell the world about your goals**

   Your friends and colleagues will ask you how the training is going and you will want to feel good about what you say – excuses are always transparent!

7. **Read as many fitness books and magazines as possible**

   They will give you new training ideas to spice up your programme.

8. **Take on public physical challenges (road races etc)**

   They will provide a training focus and the cocktail of wanting to do well mixed with the fear of public failure is always a potent motivator.

9. **Listen to other people's advice about fitness**

   They will undoubtedly give you a new perspective on exercise.

10. **Treat yourself for good behaviour**

    Though it is best to avoid three-day booze-ups and all-you-can-eat buffets.

THE MERVILLE BATTERY RAID

Achieving the impossible through daring and determination

The Normandy landings, a combined airborne and amphibious military operation that led to the liberation of France, were a key turning point in World War II. During the planning of Operation *Overlord*, it was realized that the proximity of the selected landing points to the Merville Battery constituted a significant risk. This heavily fortified German coastal artillery battery had the potential to inflict a large number of Allied casualties and even unhinge the entire operation. The battery housed four heavy artillery guns within 7ft concrete bunkers, which were protected by a mix of minefields, barbed wire fences and 130 German soldiers. The concrete bunkers that encased the guns meant that they could only be destroyed by an unlikely direct hit from the heaviest of ordnance or by a high-risk ground assault. On 6 June 1944, the task of destroying the Merville Battery fell to 9th Battalion, the Parachute Regiment, commanded by Lieutenant Colonel Terrence Otway.

The daring 9 PARA plan involved four men being inserted, ahead of the main force, to recce the target and clear paths through the surrounding perimeter and minefields. The main assault would be preceded by a barrage of 4,000lb bombs dropped from Lancaster and Halifax bombers at 0030hrs. The 650 men of 9 PARA would then have four hours from landing at their nearby drop zone to assault and secure the heavily defended position by 0500hrs, in order to prevent it from taking part in the coastal defence. Despite meticulous planning and exhaustive rehearsal the 9 PARA attack did not go according to plan. Due a combination of navigational errors, low clouds and unforeseen problems 9 PARA were scattered up to ten miles from their drop zone. By 0300hrs only 100 of the 650 men had assembled at the RV point; most notably absent were the jeeps, anti-tank guns, mortars, mine detectors, medical personnel and engineers. Another critical blow was that the RAF bombers had dropped their bombs well short of their target, causing no damage to the artillery guns. However, the advance party had performed their role brilliantly, conducting a thorough reconnaissance of the target

The rear of Merville Battery's Casemate 1 – the largest of the four gun batteries that had to be seized by 9 PARA.

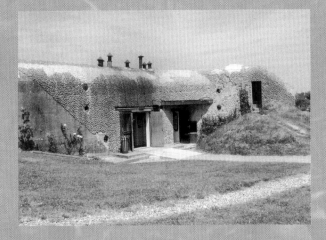

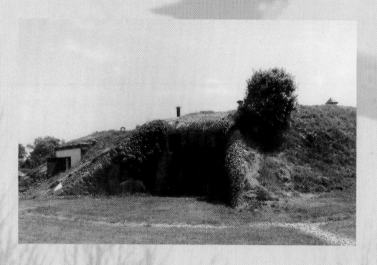

The front of Merville Battery's Casemate 1 which faced out towards Sword Beach – one of the main landing points on D-Day.

and clearing what would prove to be four vital paths through the German defence perimeter and minefields.

In true airborne spirit, Lieutenant Colonel Otway, knowing that the fate of the lives of thousands of Allied soldiers depended on 9 PARA completing its mission, redistributed his men and gave the order that the battalion (now less than one-sixth of its strength) would proceed with the men and equipment they had. Though subjected to intense enemy fire and landmine explosions, 9 PARA launched into the German stronghold with the ferocity that has become synonymous with airborne forces. The Germans held all the advantages – superior numbers and equipment and the occupation of a heavily defended position. However, 9 PARA realizing the high Allied costs associated with failure, overpowered them through guile and relentless determination. In the final stages of the battle, the paratroopers, who had expended all of their ammunition, were forced to engage the Germans in hand-to-hand fighting in order to secure their objective. By 0500hrs, 9 PARA, at the cost of 65 men either dead or seriously injured, had control of the Merville Battery and had successfully prevented it from firing upon the Normandy beaches.

In the PARAS we live by our regimental motto, *Utrinque Paratus* – 'Ready for Anything'. The 9 PARA Merville Battery raid illustrates how an approach instilled during training is translated to the battlefield. Put more simply, it was a combination of daring and bloody-minded determination that enabled 9 PARA to succeed.

I believe much can be learnt from accounts such as this one. Whether battling against a fierce enemy, or against mental and physical barriers which prevent you from accomplishing the things you want to achieve, the decisive battle takes place in your mind – and to win you must believe that the rewards that come with success outweigh the cost of attaining them!

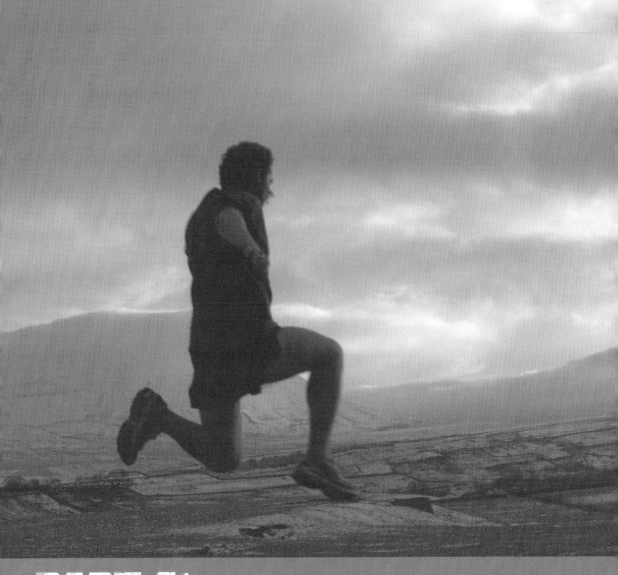

PART 4:
STANDARD OPERATING
PROCEDURES

'The successful person has the habit of doing the things failures don't like to do. They don't like doing them either necessarily. But their disliking is subordinated to the strength of their purpose.'

E.M. Gray

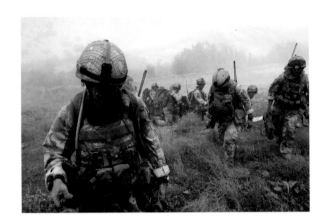

As well as reacting to UK military emergencies overseas, the Parachute Regiment also routinely deploys on six-month operations, most recently in Iraq and Afghanistan. While these operations rarely involve parachuting, they are still dangerous. Immediately before and after these deployments we go through a period of consolidation in order to either prepare for or unwind from the operation. Experience has proved that prior preparation is vital to the success of our operations, while the decompression phase is every bit as important to our success on subsequent operations. Our mandatory preparatory training provides us with the time, focus and environment to develop our tactics at individual and group levels. We start slowly, but gradually increase the intensity until our preparation includes similar stress levels to those we will face on the operation. The training not only develops our skills, but focuses our minds and forges us as a team. Without pre-deployment training, we run the risk of suffering numerous casualties in the early stages of our tour as we acclimatize to the challenges that face us in our new environment. This acclimatization is every bit as important after the tour. Having experienced unique levels of stress, hardship and anxiety we then have to adapt to the routines of life with our families and friends, of whom few could understand what we have been through. Decompression provides a safe environment to reflect on the past six months together and resolve any issues before resuming our lives back at home.

In a similar way, physical exercise puts the body under a level of stress and exertion it does not encounter in normal daily life. If exercise is tackled from a standing start, the body struggles to cope with the new demands being placed on it and, in many cases, our connective tissues fail and injury is the result. Having worked the body at a high tempo, it is equally important to undergo a process of gradually cooling the body down after exercise, without which the first casualty is the subsequent session.

Warming Up

The warm-up is a key part of any training session. It is designed to raise the body's temperature and prepare the mind and body for vigorous activity. Research suggests that the optimum warm-up duration, before undertaking stretching activities, is 15 minutes. However, it is possible to achieve an adequate effect from around 5 minutes. The warm-up should consist of a gradual increase in intensity until the heart is working at 70% of its maximum. A warm-up at this intensity has the effect of allowing an increase in the range of movement of the joints and improving aerobic performance. The body becomes more flexible and exercise efficiency improves. Warm-ups should be split into a first and second pulse raiser, one before stretching and the other after.

A warm-up produces a 2–3°C rise in body temperature, leading to beneficial changes in body tissue:

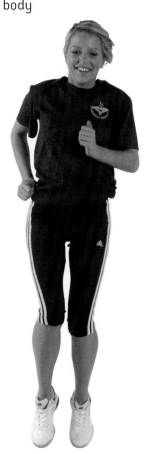

- The heating effect allows muscles and tendons to become more flexible and reduces the risk of muscle strains.
- There is an increase in blood flow, which means that there is an increase in the flow of oxygen to muscle tissue.
- There is an increase in blood temperature enabling more oxygen to enter the muscle tissue.
- The increase in temperature improves the efficiency of muscle contraction through increased enzyme and metabolic activity.
- During the second pulse raiser, exercise-specific activities activate neural pathways and speed up the body's reaction time.

In addition to the physiological effects, the warm-up has the effect of preparing you psychologically by encouraging you to focus on the physical activity to follow.

FIRST PULSE RAISER

The purpose of the first pulse raiser is to increase circulation to your major muscle groups. It should last around five minutes. The activity should be similar in intensity to a quick walk or light jog.

Find a safe area to gradually progress from a walk into a light jog. Once jogging, perform each of the activities below; as well as increasing your pulse rate they will also help mobilize your joints. If you lack space in your exercise area all of these activities can be performed from a static position.

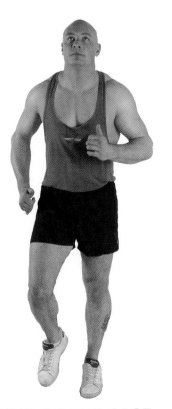

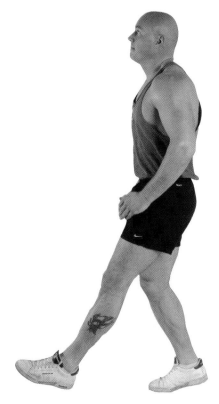

JOGGING ON THE SPOT

Replicate the arm and shoulder movement of running, without forward motion.

CALF KICKS

While jogging, exaggerate the forward movement of each stride, pointing your toes forward and leaning back slightly.

HEEL RAISES

While jogging, exaggerate the rearward motion of each stride, aiming to get your heels progressively closer to your bottom.

HIGH KNEES

While jogging, move on to the balls of your feet and exaggerate the forward motion of each stride by gradually bringing your knees higher until they are parallel with your waist.

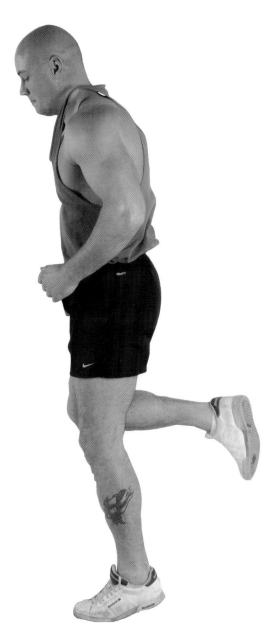
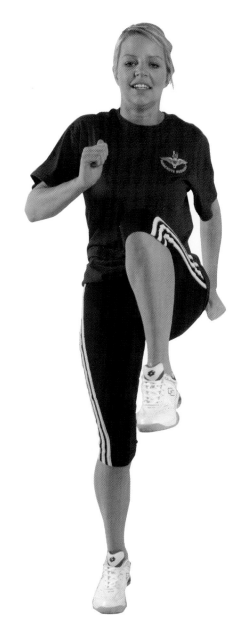

Stretching

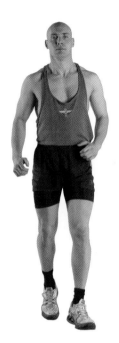

As we have heard, extensive research suggests that performing a warm-up and a cool-down before and after activity can help reduce the incidence of injury and promote recovery following training. A key part of these is improving flexibility through stretching. In order to understand correct stretching techniques, it is important to first know about some of the biochemical and physiological properties of the soft tissues that you are stretching.

All soft tissues (muscles, tendons, joint capsules) are more flexible when they are warm. All stretching is ineffective if it is performed when the body is cold, and should, therefore, be preceded by a series of warm-up exercises to increase tissue temperature, hence the purpose of the first pulse raiser.

All muscles and tendons have a neural reflex which prevents hyperextension. Nerves within the muscle are sensitive to changes in muscle length and tension. When a muscle is stretched, the muscle sends a message to the central nervous system to cause a reflex contraction of the muscle in order to prevent stretch damage. However, if the stretch is maintained for more than six seconds, the nerve responds by sending a signal to the central nervous system which causes the muscle to relax. This is why all stretches should be done slowly with a gradual increase in the range of movement. Stretches can be categorized as follows:

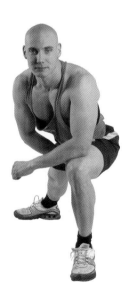

SIMPLE STRETCH

A simple stretch is typically used when recovering from injuries, rather than when fit. During the stretch you should feel a very mild tension in the muscle. Simple stretches should be held for 10–30 seconds.

DEVELOPMENTAL STRETCH

A developmental stretch is the main type of stretch used before and after exercise. When stretching you should feel a tension, which then disappears after about 15 seconds. If it doesn't disappear, you are stretching too hard and risk injuring yourself. Developmental stretches should be held for 20–30 seconds. Mobility exercises should be done before exercising.

MOBILITY EXERCISES

The purpose of these exercises is to get your joints to move more freely prior to stretching and exercise.

NECK MOBILITY >

Stand up straight. Now turn your head to the left until your chin is over your shoulder, hold for 3–5 seconds, then do the same on the right-hand side. Repeat this exercise three times on both sides. Now bend your head forward until your chin is as close to your chest as possible, hold for 3–5 seconds, then lean your head backwards as far as is comfortable and hold for 3–5 seconds. Repeat this exercise three times.

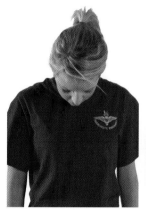

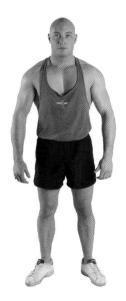
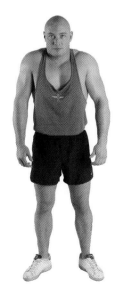

< SHOULDER MOBILITY

Stand with your feet shoulder-width apart and your shoulder muscles relaxed. Now, contracting your shoulder and back muscles, raise your shoulders as high as possible and hold for 3–5 seconds. Repeat this exercise three times.

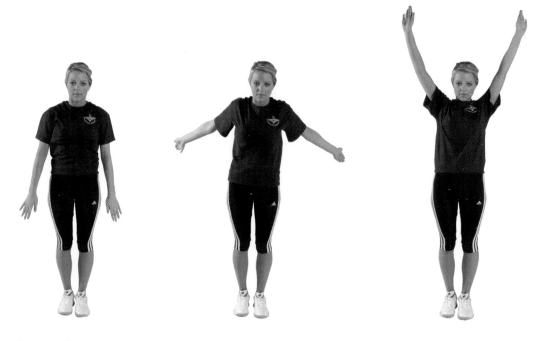

ARM MOBILITY ∧

Stand facing forwards with your legs together and your arms fully extended by your sides. Now, keeping your arms straight, rotate your arms forwards, aiming to keep your arms straight so that they lightly rub against your legs and ears as they pass them. Complete five forward rotations, followed by five backward rotations.

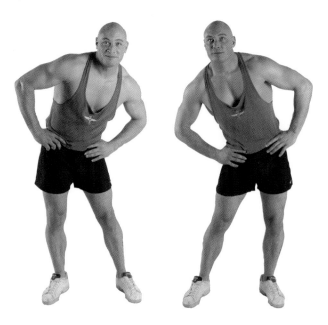

< HIP MOBILITY

Stand with your feet shoulder-width apart and your hands on your hips. Now, make five clockwise followed by five anti-clockwise rotations with your hips, as if you are balancing a hula hoop around your waist.

DEVELOPMENTAL STRETCHES

As described earlier, stretching is designed to prepare your muscles for vigorous exercise, by mobilizing specific muscle and connective tissue groups.

ARMS AND SHOULDERS STRETCH >

Stand with your feet shoulder-width apart, interlock your fingers with your palms facing in, tense your arms, and push your hands as far away from your chest as possible. Hold this stretch for 10–15 seconds.

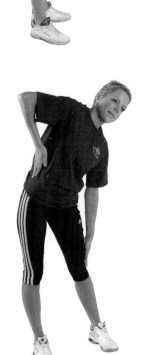

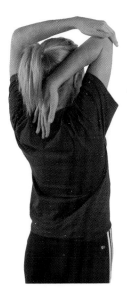

< TRICEP STRETCH

While standing, place your right palm on the top of your spine with your elbow pointing to the sky; now, using your left hand, push down on your right elbow towards your spine, until you feel the stretch in your tricep. Hold the stretch for 10–15 seconds and repeat on your left arm.

TRUNK STRETCH >

Stand facing forwards with your feet shoulder-width apart, keeping your neck and back straight. Lean to your left, using your left arm to reach as far down your left leg as is comfortable. Hold for 10–15 seconds, then repeat on your right side.

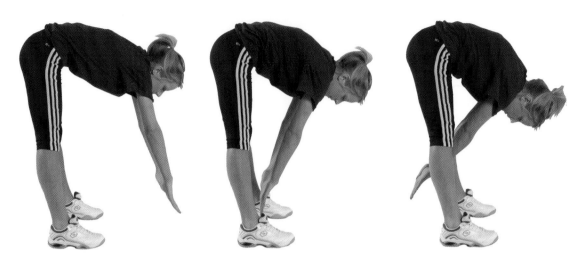

HAMSTRING STRETCH ∧

Stand with your legs about 60cm/2ft apart. Keeping your arms straight, bend forwards and reach towards the ground in front of you, and hold for 10–15 seconds. Now repeat the exercise, reaching for a point on the ground between your legs, and then behind your legs.

CALF STRETCH >

1. In a modified press-up position, with your buttocks higher than your head, anchor the ball of your left foot on the floor and use your weight to push your left heel towards the floor until you feel the stretch. Trail your spare foot around the back of your ankle. Hold for 10–15 seconds and repeat on both sides. To increase the stretch, increase the space between your hands and feet.

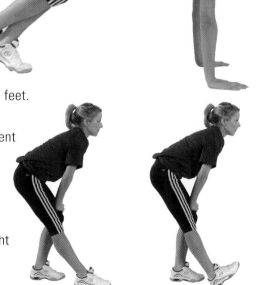

2. Stand with your right leg straight, your left leg bent and your knees together. Keeping both feet on the floor, lean forwards and place both arms on your bent leg. To feel the stretch push your buttocks backwards and towards the ground. To increase the intensity of the stretch, raise the toes of your straight leg. Hold for 10–15 seconds and repeat on the opposite leg.

QUAD STRETCH >

Stand with your back and neck straight. Bend your right knee, bringing your foot to your buttocks, while holding the laces of your right shoe. Keep your knees together and push forward with your hips to increase the intensity of the stretch. Hold for 10–15 seconds and repeat on the opposite leg.

PARTNER QUAD STRETCH

If struggling to maintain balance, either find a partner or a fixed object to aid balance. Use the opposite arm to that holding your laces to support yourself. (See page 93.)

GROIN STRETCH ∨

Sit on the floor and place the heels of your feet together in front of you. While holding your ankles, use your elbows to push your knees towards the ground. Hold for 10–15 seconds.

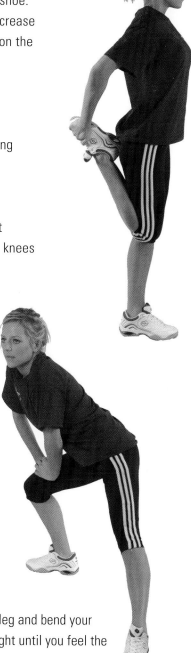

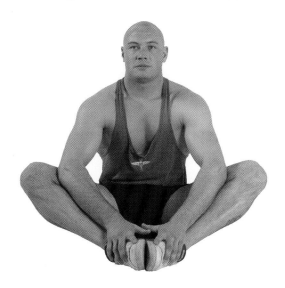

INNER THIGH STRETCH >

Stand with your feet parallel about 1m/3ft apart. Extend your left leg and bend your right knee. Place both hands on your right knee and lean to your right until you feel the stretch in your inner thigh. Hold for 10–15 seconds and repeat on the opposite side.

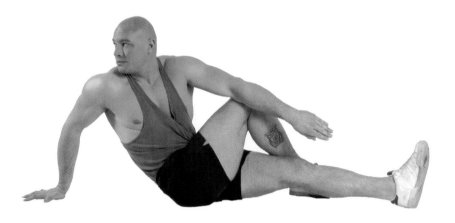

BUTTOCKS

Sit on the floor with your legs outstretched. Place your right foot so that the outside of your right foot is next to the outside of your left knee and your right knee points up towards the sky. Supporting your body with your right arm, use the elbow of your left arm to push against the outside of your right knee until you feel the stretch in your buttocks. Hold for 10–15 seconds and repeat on the opposite side.

SECOND PULSE RAISER

The final part of your warm-up is the second pulse raiser. Your muscles and joints should now be mobile and warm. The aim of the second pulse raiser is to prepare your body to commence exercise. It should last 3–5 minutes and replicate the type and intensity of your exercise session. For example a running session should be preceded by a 3–5 minute running pulse raiser, just as a warm-up prior to circuit training should include some circuit training exercises. At the end of your warm-up you should feel ready to start your workout.

Cooling Down

The purpose of a cool-down is to optimise recovery after activity. During exercise the body is put under stress, which leads to an increase in body temperature, heart rate and blood pressure. Another by-product of exercise is the release of hormones, such as adrenaline and endorphins, into the circulatory system. If you stop exercising suddenly, the adrenaline and endorphin levels in your system can result in feelings of restlessness and even a sleepless night. Equally, waste products such as lactic acid are thought to cause tiredness and stiffness. The cool-down, therefore, not only prevents a rapid decrease in body temperature, heart rate and blood pressure, but actively remove waste products by gently working the major muscle groups. At the same time your body also releases hormones to counter the effects of adrenaline and allow rest and sleep after exercise. Due to the body's heightened temperature, this is a perfect time to stretch and enhance your flexibility. You should aim to spend at least ten minutes cooling down.

PULSE REDUCTION

Spend a couple of minutes walking at a moderate pace. Your goal here is to gradually reduce your heart rate and control your circulation.

STRETCHING

Now follow exactly the same set of stretches you performed during your warm-up, but this time hold each stretch for 20–25 seconds. Your goal here is not only to prevent muscle stiffness, but to increase the flexibility of your muscles while they are warm.

THE 2 PARA FALKLANDS VOYAGE

Training with limited resources: 'Necessity is the mother of innovation.'

The Falkland Islands, a small group of islands in the South Atlantic, emerged from obscurity in 1982, after they were invaded by Argentina. When diplomatic efforts failed to reach a peaceful resolution to the invasion, the UK responded by assembling a task force to regain control of the islands. This task force included 2 and 3 PARA. 2 PARA were recalled from leave and within a couple of days all 550 soldiers were sailing towards the Falklands on the North Sea ferry MV *Norland*. In the following four weeks, this holiday ship was transformed into a floating gymnasium to prepare the battalion for what would face them at Goose Green. When 2 PARA set sail from Southampton they didn't know that they would have to TAB the length of the island carrying Bergens weighing in excess of 120lbs, before defeating an Argentinian force nearly three times their size. Fortunately, for those four weeks this is exactly what 2 PARA prepared for.

Recalled from leave, the men of 2 PARA embarked on the MV *Norland* and sailed from Portsmouth on 26 April 1982.

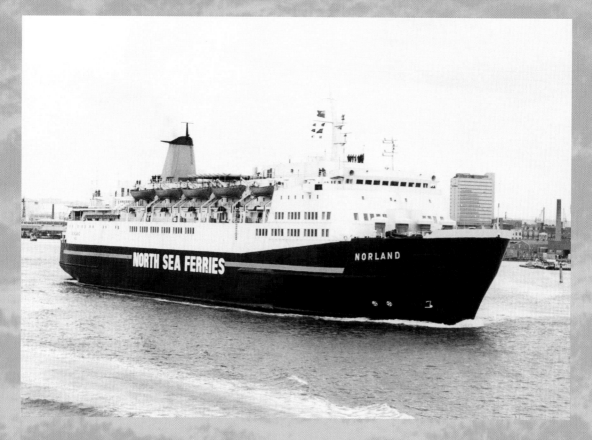

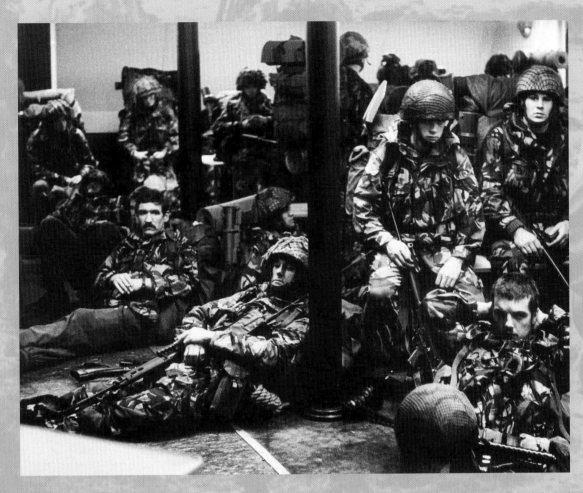

Fitness became a twice-daily ritual for the 2 PARA soldiers. The PARA physical training instructors (PTIs) were tasked with devising a progressive programme, which worked with the limited equipment and space available, to get rid of the excesses of an extended leave period and prepare the battalion for its most demanding task since World War II. In 1982, the fitness revolution had yet to gain momentum, and what exercise facilities the *Norland* had were inadequate for 550 paratroopers preparing for war. The PTIs, therefore, had to resort to the basics; body to weight exercises (pull-ups, press-ups etc), improvised weights, shuttle runs, circuit training, fireman's carries and battle marches were all that were on offer. Each company of 120 men assembled both morning and afternoon on the hastily constructed flight deck for two two-hour fitness sessions. At first, the fitness sessions revolved around moderate runs and light circuit training

After a month of intense training at sea, the men of 2 PARA wait on board the *Norland* before the landings at San Carlos.

exercises, but as the voyage progressed so did the intensity of the exercises, until the soldiers were parading in full battle order to run continuously around the deck. Alongside the compulsory exercise programmes, numerous fitness competitions were devised at section, platoon and individual level to ignite the natural competitiveness of paratroopers. Fitness was not only a means of conditioning their minds and bodies for the challenges ahead but, along with the other technical skills that were being taught, it provided each soldier with a focus and alleviated the boredom between meal times.

With a clear goal and a programme that gradually increased the frequency and intensity of their physical activity, 2 PARA achieved a fitness level in four weeks that university sports science students won't come close to in three years. They arrived at the Falklands in June in possibly the best physical shape they had ever been in. This had been accomplished in spite of the limited resources at their disposal, not because of them. But as has been found on the battlefield many times over, the resources that really count are determination and the will to win.

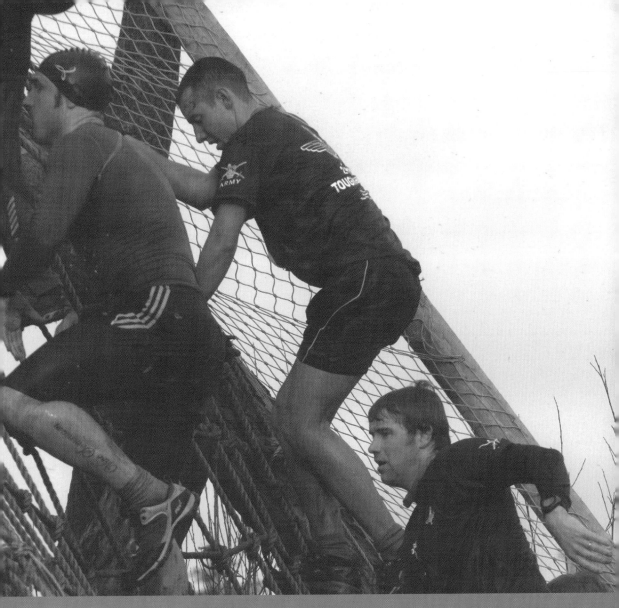

PART 5:
THE P COMPANY SPARTAN
PROGRAMME (NO FRILLS)

'The fight is won or lost far away from witnesses – behind the lines, in the gym, and out there on the road, long before I dance under those lights.'

Muhammad Ali

As described in Part 1, paratroopers need to be prepared for anything. This means being equipped with the mental and physical fitness to deal with every foreseeable challenge they might face on the battlefield. The Parachute Regiment's success depends on it. Every paratrooper must be equipped with the strength and endurance to carry a heavy pack over a harrowing insertion march, and still have the speed and resilience to shock and overpower his enemy in the assault. PARA fitness matches the demands made on PARAS, and PARA training focuses on getting recruits to achieve this blend and level of fitness. Paratroopers are not trained to win marathons, nor are they trained for power lifting. PARA training develops strength, speed, endurance and flexibility alongside each other, rather than in isolation. In doing so, it delivers paratroopers who have both the physical and mental capacity to stay on top in the most challenging of environments, not just on the athletics track.

With this programme, all you will need is the bare essentials of sports kit, and the determination and perseverance to see the

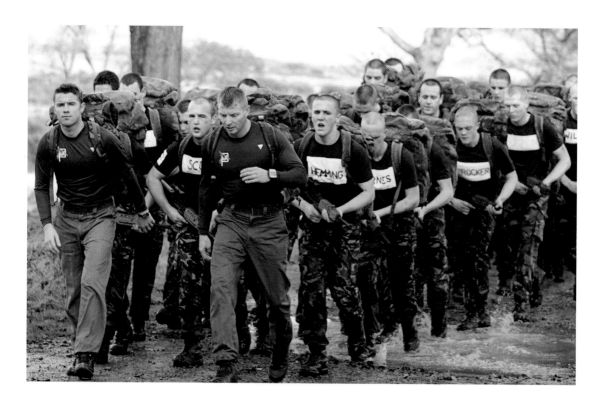

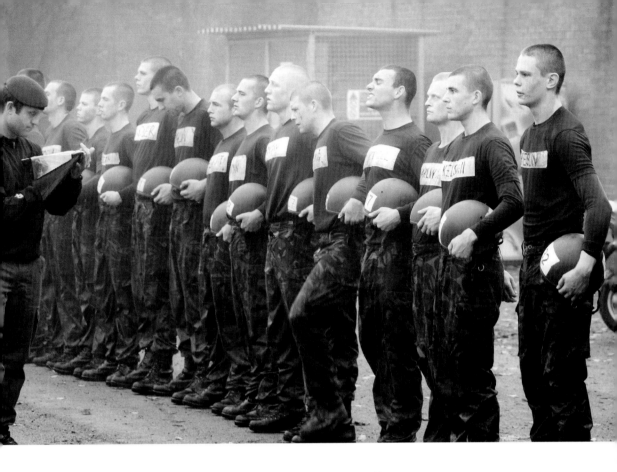

programme through. As was illustrated perfectly by 2 PARA's voyage to the Falklands, you don't need state-of-the-art gym equipment, or acres of sports fields, to get into supreme physical shape. The ingredients that this programme is based on can easily be found in immediate proximity to your home. This gritty approach has been directly inspired by our PARA programme; a training process which has been refined continually over the last 70 years to make us one of the fiercest fighting forces in the world.

Each of the three programmes has been tailored to develop your fitness, starting at the level you are at now. Within each programme there is the scope to taper the intensity of your session to your ability, but the intention is for you to gradually take each programme as a stepping stone to achieving your fitness goal. Like PARA training, no assumptions are made. Using a combination of the advice on running and circuit training and the exercise descriptions provided in Part 4, nothing is left to chance. Incremental and progressive, this programme will be crawl, walk, run. However, I promise in no time it will feel like you are sprinting. Your pilgrimage to PARA fitness starts now!

Running

As a species, our ability to run has enabled us to survive and, therefore, we have been running ever since we first existed. However, to get the best results it is important to use specific training sessions to increase your body's capacity to run faster and for longer. No more junk miles!

INTERVAL TRAINING

Interval training, as the name suggests, involves training at a specific intensity for a sustained period, followed by a rest, followed by repeating this process a number of times. Interval training is an extremely effective method of training and works by overloading the body and educating it on what it feels like to run quicker than it is used to. Interval sessions are measured by distance (e.g. 200m or between four lamp posts). If you're new to interval training, you will definitely find it quite hard – the trick is to build up slowly. Fartlek is an example of interval training.

FARTLEK TRAINING

In Fartlek training you vary the speed at which you are running at different stages of a run, so for set periods of time you will run at fast, slow and sometimes intermediate paces. Fartlek works by increasing your body's capacity to deal with lactic acid, a by-product of intense exercise. Fartlek training switches between steady state and fast running, which not only means anyone can do it, but also that it is always a challenging session. You can gradually increase the Fartlek session by upping the pace, or length, of the fast intervals in relation to the rest periods.

HILL REPS

Hill reps are a type of interval training that achieve periods of increased exercise intensity by selecting steeper gradients for a predetermined

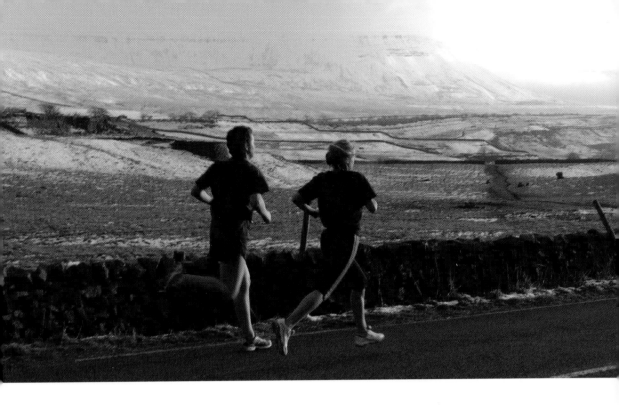

number of burst repetitions, interspersed with periods of rest. The gradient, duration and rest between repetitions can be adjusted to make the session more or less demanding.

THRESHOLD RUNNING

Threshold or tempo running, as the name suggests, involves running at your aerobic threshold (as fast as possible while still running aerobically) for a continuous period. This type of training session works by gradually increasing the pace and duration at which your body can deal with the lactic acid produced during exertion. It is best to progress slowly into tempo running by either starting slowly, or breaking your run into phases; like an interval session, but with less difference between the interval paces.

RECOVERY RUN

A recovery run is a slow run designed to allow the body to get rid of the waste products from previous sessions. This type of run is normally done by endurance runners after a competition, or during a period of intense training. It is important to ensure that recovery runs don't turn into junk miles. The aim of these runs is to flush out waste products, not add unnecessary miles to your training programme.

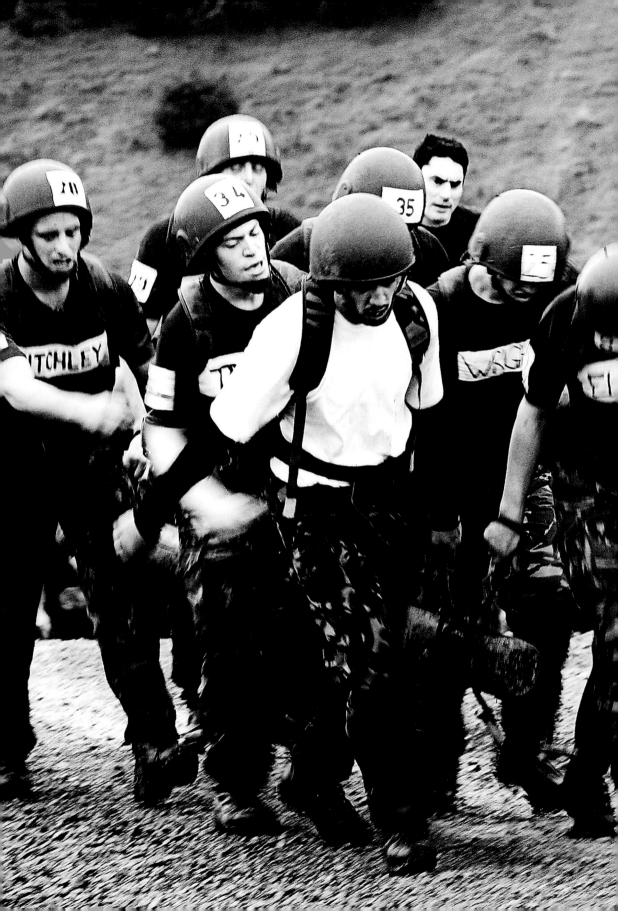

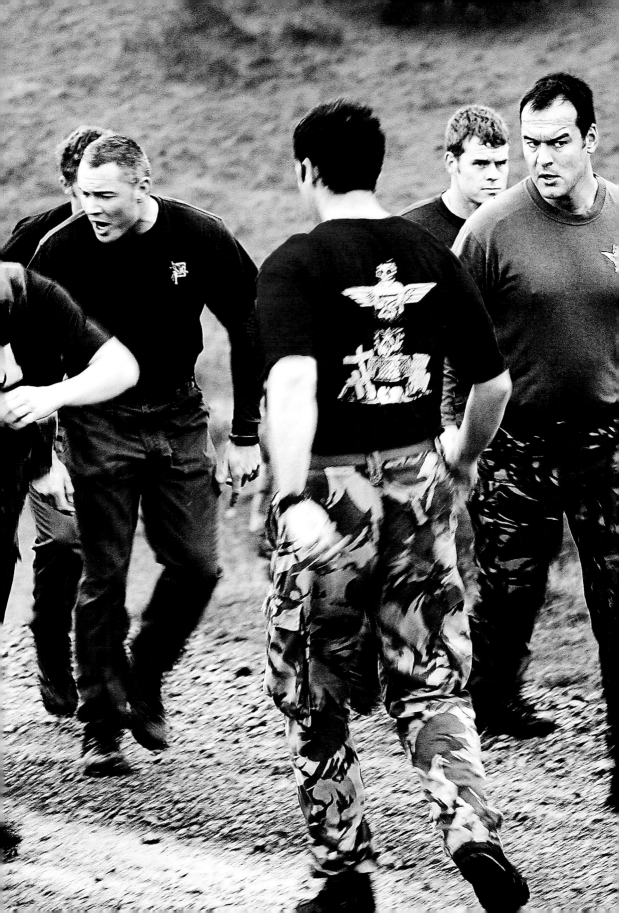

Circuit Training

Circuit training is the name given to a group of strength exercises that are completed one exercise after another, with each exercise being performed for a specified number of repetitions, or for a prescribed period of time, before moving on to the next exercise. It forms a large part of the paratrooper training programme because it is an excellent way to improve all aspects of personal fitness. Circuit training has a number of advantages when compared to other forms of exercise:

- It develops both strength and muscular endurance at the same time.
- It can be tailored to most sports and varying fitness and health levels.
- It can be conducted effectively without the use of specialized fitness equipment.
- It is easy for a newcomer, or recent returner to exercise to create a good circuit session themselves.

The total number and type of circuit exercises performed during a training session can be changed to fit your ability, the time available for training, or your training goal. As well as using the examples given in each of the training programmes detailed in this book, it is really easy to set up your own circuit training session. It is easy to tailor your session to a specific fitness goal, but a general circuit training session will normally include a circuit of exercises performed for a number of rotations. It is common to rest for a set period between each exercise and alternate between leg, trunk and upper body exercises, although some exercises, such as burpees, involve all three.

In each circuit it is important not to have consecutive exercises using the same muscle group. To make it easier to remember what exercise you are going to do next, either write your programme down, or create cards to be placed where you intend to do each exercise. You can alter the number of repetitions you do of each exercise along with the total number of circuits you do, but a session would typically include:

- Warm-up.
- A form circuit typically the second pulse raiser (e.g. 15 seconds per exercise).
- 3–4 incremental circuits, which are time or repetition based (e.g. 30, 45, 60 seconds per exercise or 10, 20, 30 repetitions per exercise).
- Rest for 15 seconds between each exercise and for 2–3 minutes between each complete circuit.
- Cool-down.

CIRCUIT TRAINING EXERCISES

In Part 4 I was serving a set meal, but in this section I give you a menu for you to choose from according to your appetite for challenge and progress. I have broken down the circuit training exercises by the area of the body they work on. You will find that within each sub-section the exercises get progressively more difficult. In the training programmes at the end of this chapter, you will see that your programme does not specify which type of activity you should do during your session. Instead the idea is that as you get fitter, you include progressively more demanding exercises as part of your training programme.

EXERCISE LEVEL SYMBOLS

 Recruit level: suitable for beginners

 Soldier level: suitable for those with an intermediate level of fitness

 Paratrooper level: the ultimate test, suitable for those who have reached peak fitness

No symbol indicates that the exercise is suitable for all fitness levels

PRESS-UPS

Press-ups are a brilliant way to exercise your arms, back, chest and abs. I have included seven different types of press-up, starting with the easiest and getting progressively more difficult.

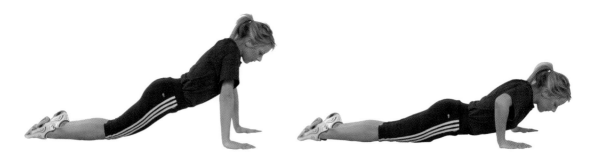

KNEE PRESS-UPS

From all fours, place your hands shoulder-width apart so that your arms are fully extended and your feet and knees are on the floor. Now, lower your body until your chest and hips are about an inch from the floor, making sure you keep your neck and back straight. Then fully extend your arms until you return to your start position.

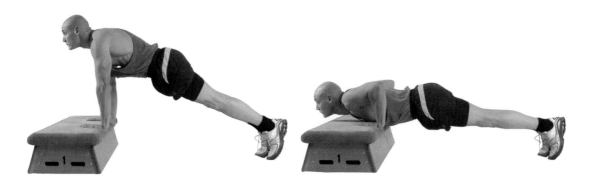

INCLINE PRESS-UPS

Start from a traditional press-up position – back straight with your arms shoulder-width apart – but rest your hands on a raised surface (the lower the incline the more difficult it will be). Now, keeping your back straight, lower your body until your chest and hips are about an inch from the floor.

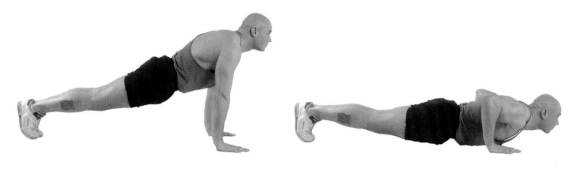

STANDARD PRESS-UP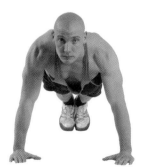

With your arms fully extended shoulder-width apart, your back straight, and your hands and feet on the floor, lower your body until your chest and hips are about an inch from the floor.

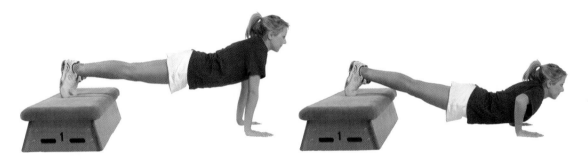

DECLINE PRESS-UP

For a decline press-up, do a standard press-up, but with your feet on a raised surface – the higher the surface the more difficult it will be.

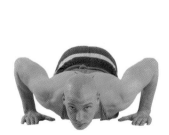
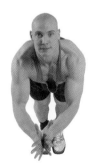

CLAP PRESS-UP

From the standard press-up position, lower your chest and hips until they are about an inch from the floor, then extend your arms with sufficient power to clap between each repetition.

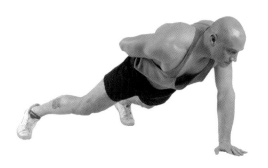
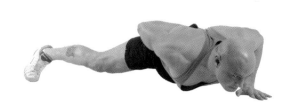

ONE-ARM PRESS-UP

Adopt a standard press-up position, but fold one arm behind your back. Now, using your extended arm, lower your chest and hips until they are about an inch from the floor.

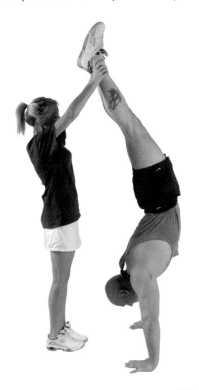
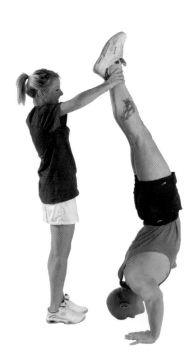

HANDSTAND PRESS-UPS

With a partner standing in front of you to hold your legs or using a wall for support, move into a handstand with your hands shoulder-width apart. Keeping your back and legs straight, use your arms to lower your head to the ground then straighten your arms until they are fully extended. The handstand press-up is the most difficult type of press-up, and it mainly exercises the upper arms.

DIPS

The following dips require either access to a purpose-built dip bar or some kind of improvisation. In the past, I have used the tops of two sturdy chairs back to back (seats facing outwards) but this is a much less comfortable or sturdy means of performing dips than using a specially designed dip bar.

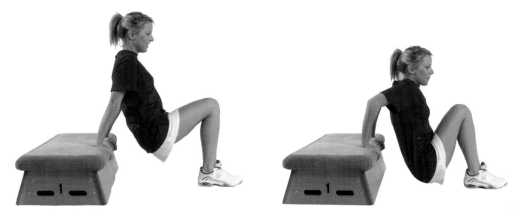

BENCH DIPS 🔺

With your legs bent and your feet on the floor, place your hands behind you on a surface raised about 1–2ft higher than your feet. Now lower your body with your arms until your buttocks are about an inch from the floor.

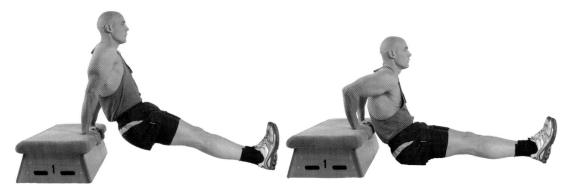

BENCH DIPS 🔺

With your legs fully extended in front of you and your arms on a surface 1–2ft above your feet, lower your buttocks until they are about an inch from the floor.

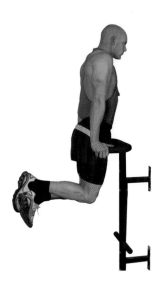
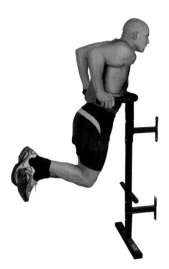

TRADITIONAL DIPS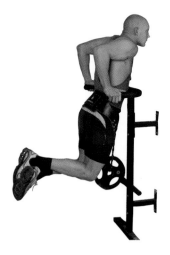

With your arms fully extended and supporting your weight, and your knees bent, lower your body until your arms are parallel with the floor. Now use your arms to return to your start position.

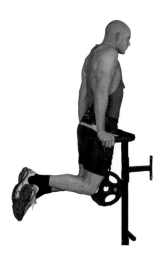
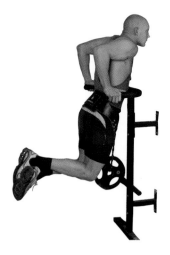

WEIGHTED DIP

For a weighted dip, you need to find a suitable weight to increase the intensity of your exercise. This would typically be a weight belt attached to a free weight; however, I have used a small rucksack filled with water (preventing the rucksack from interfering with your arm movement is key). With your arms fully extended and supporting your weight, and your knees bent, lower your body with your arms until arms are parallel with the floor. Now use your arms to return to your start position.

PULL-UPS

Pull-ups are the king of body to weight exercises. While it is easiest to do this exercise on a specially designed bar, I have used everything from door frames to bus shelters. All you need is a ledge to hold on to and nothing underneath. I have included four different pull-up variants, starting with the easiest.

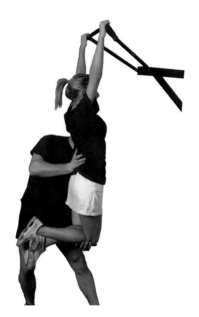
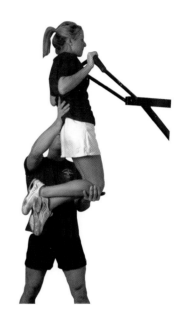

ASSISTED PULL-UPS

Either using a specific pull-up machine, or with the aid of a partner, take hold of the pull-up bar and fully extend your arms. Now pull your body up until your chin is over the bar, keeping your feet together and your knees bent throughout.

As an intermediate step between assisted pull-ups and the real thing, try lowering yourself unassisted between each repetition.

Tips on assisting: It is important to assist rather than do the work for your partner; as a rule you should not be taking any more than 25% of the weight. Place one arm at the base of your partner's spine and the other under both knees. This will prevent your partner falling forward if they let go of the bar.

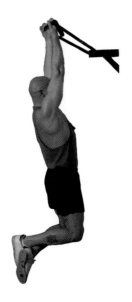
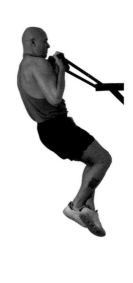

UNDERARM PULL-UP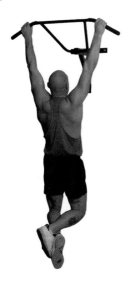

Take hold of the bar using an underarm grip and fully extend your arms. Now use your arms to lift your body up until your chin is raised above the bar, keeping your feet tight together and your legs bent throughout.

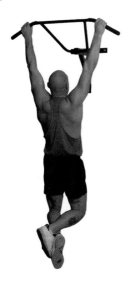
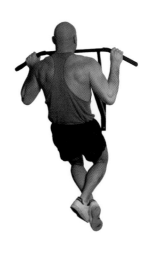

OVERARM PULL-UP

For the overarm pull-up the only thing that changes is your grip. Grasp the bar with an overhand grip with arms fully extended, then lift your body until your chin is raised above the bar.

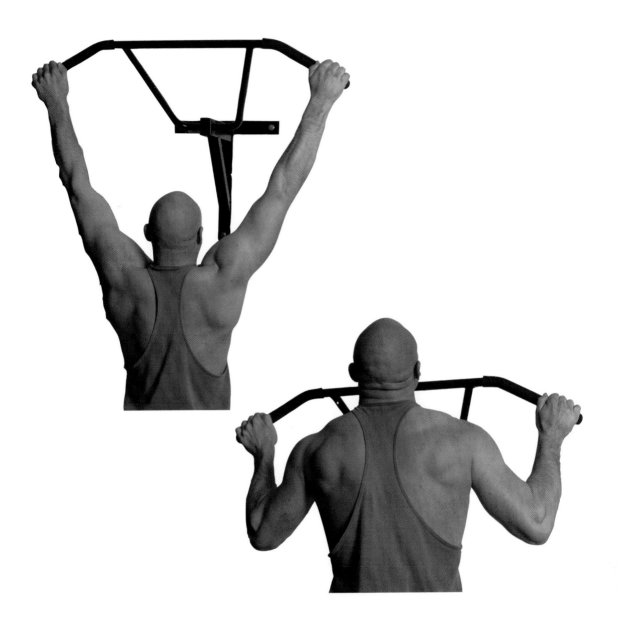

WIDE ARM PULL-UP 🏋

This is a variation of the overarm pull-up, this time with a wider grip, which isolates your shoulder muscles more. With your arms fully extended, lift your body until your chin is over the bar.

ABS

Sit-ups are a tried and tested exercise for training and toning abs. They require no specialist equipment, but a mat or towel to lie on can certainly improve your comfort while exercising. I have included six variations of the sit-up and they get progressively more difficult.

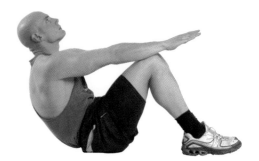

HALF SIT-UP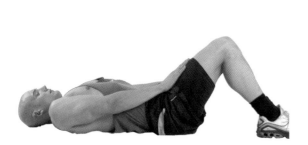

Lie on your back with your legs bent and the palms of your hands on your thighs. Using your stomach muscles, reach forward until your fully extended arms move towards your knees. The further you reach, the more difficult the exercise.

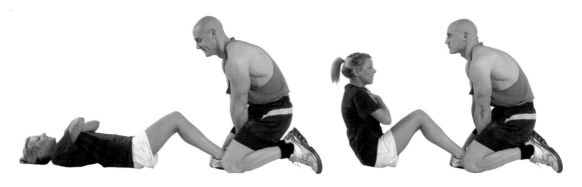

PARTNER SIT-UPS

Lie on your back with your knees bent and your arms crossed across your chest. Using a heavy object or a partner to keep your feet on the floor, contract your stomach muscles until your chest is perpendicular to the floor, then gradually release until you return to your start point.

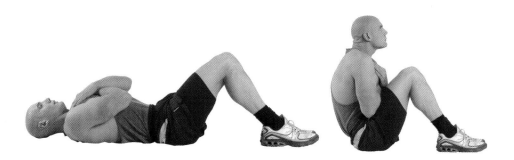

FULL SIT-UP

Lie on your back with your knees bent and your arms crossed across your chest. Now, using your stomach muscles, lift your chest until it is perpendicular to the ground, making sure your feet remain firmly on the ground. Now lower back under control and repeat.

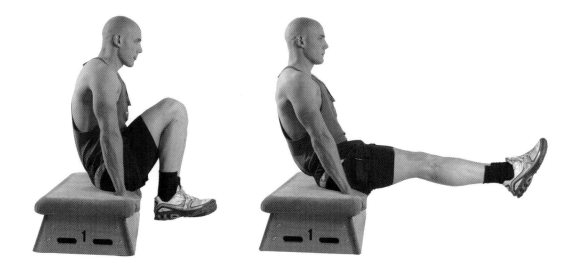

RAISED LEG EXTENSIONS

Sit on the edge of a raised surface with your knees up and your feet together off the floor. Now fully extend your legs until they are parallel with the ground, hold for one second, and then return them under control to your start position. Throughout you should use your arms to aid balance.

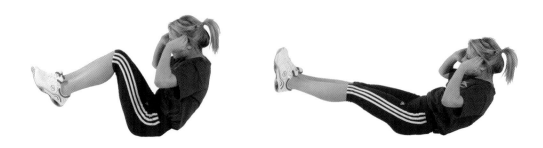

CRUNCH SIT-UP

Start with your buttocks on the floor, your legs and chest slightly raised, and your fingertips resting on your temples. Now, using your abdominal muscles and hip flexors, bring up your knees and arms until they are a couple of inches apart, then lower them under control, and repeat.

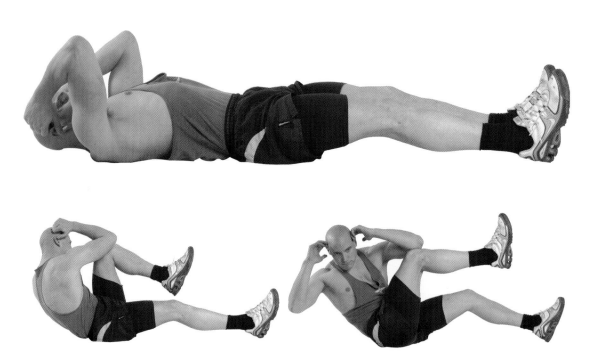

TWIST SIT-UPS

Start on your back with your legs extended and your fingers next to your temples. Now, using your abdominal muscles and hip flexors, move your right elbow to your left knee, return to your start point under control, then move your left elbow to your right knee.

CORE STABILITY

While a relatively new term, core stability is not a new concept. It relates to training your core stomach, leg and back muscles by using a series of static exercises.

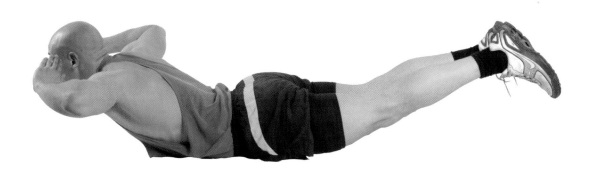

DORSAL RAISE

Lie face down on the floor, with your fingertips touching your temples. Now, lift your torso and legs off the floor at the same time and hold for 10–15 seconds before lowering under control.

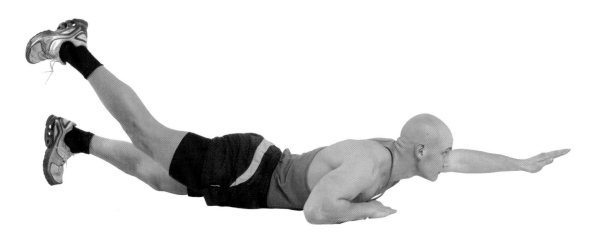

SUPERMAN

Lie face down on the floor, with your arms and legs fully extended. Now, raise opposite arms and legs together and hold off the floor for 10–15 seconds. Repeat three times on either side.

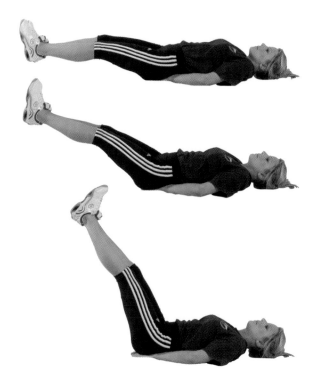

LEG RAISES

Lie on your back with your palms facing down, tucked under your buttocks. Now, keeping your legs straight, raise your feet so they are six inches, 12 inches then 18 inches off the floor, holding for 15 seconds at each level.

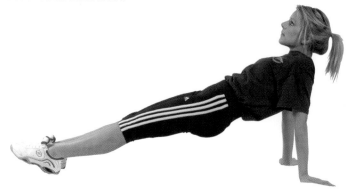

REVERSE PLANK

Resting on your heels and palms, push your hips forward so that your back is straight, and maintain this position using your abdominal muscles.

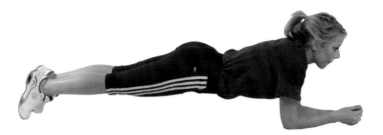

THE PLANK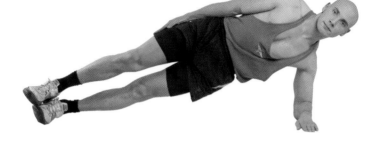

Resting on your forearms and toes, use your abdominal muscles to maintain a straight back and hold this position.

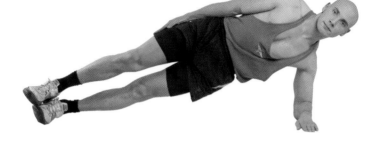

SIDE PLANK

Supporting your body on your left forearm and the side of your left foot, use your abdominal muscles to maintain a straight back and hold this position. Repeat on the other side.

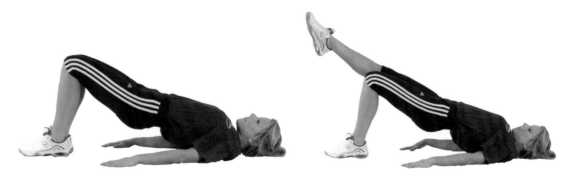

BRIDGE

Lie on the floor with your arms by your side, legs bent and your feet flat on the floor. Now, using your abs, hold your stomach up so that it is in line with your thighs. It is possible to increase the intensity of the bridge by extending one leg fully throughout the repetition.

LEG EXERCISES

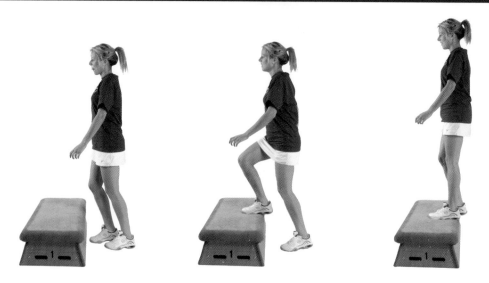

STEP-UPS

Find a raised, stable surface (the higher it is, the more difficult the exercise) and step up onto it one foot at a time until both feet are off the floor, then step down one foot after the other.

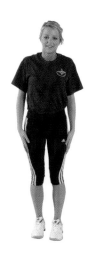
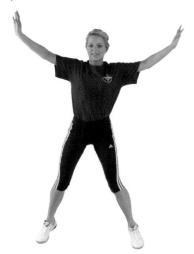

STRIDE JUMPS

Stand with your feet together and your arms by your sides. Jump so your legs are wide apart and your arms are extended, then jump back to your start position.

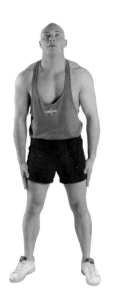
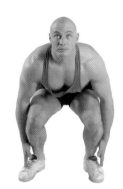
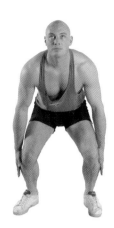

SQUATS

Stand with your feet shoulder-width apart and your arms by your sides. Bend your knees, keeping your face forward and your back straight, until your hands touch the floor at the side of each foot, then stand up under control.

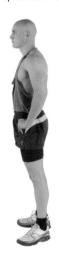
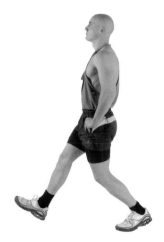
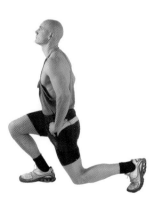

LUNGES

Stand with your feet together and your hands on your hips. Now, lunge forward with your right foot until your left knee is about two inches from the floor, then step back with your right foot until both feet are together again and repeat with the opposite foot. Keep your back straight throughout this exercise.

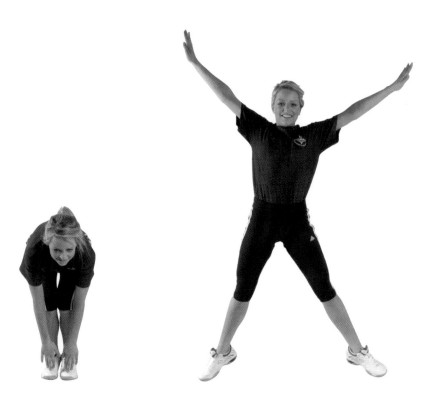

STAR JUMPS

From a crouching position, holding your feet with your hands, jump as high as you can with your arms and legs outstretched before landing back in the crouch position.

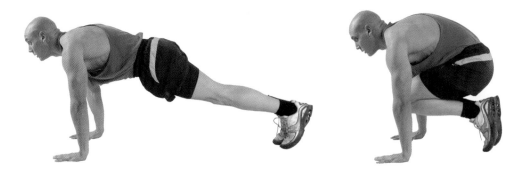

SQUAT THRUSTS

Start in the standard press-up position. Jump both legs forwards to a crouch position where your knees are in front of your elbows, then jump both legs back to the press-up position.

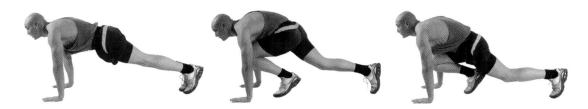

ALTERNATE SQUAT THRUSTS

Starting in the standard press-up position, thrust your left leg forwards until it is forward of your elbows, then bring your left leg back and your right knee forward of your elbows at the same time. Remain on the balls of your feet throughout the exercise.

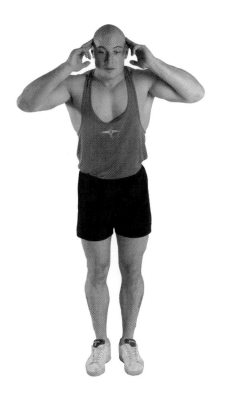

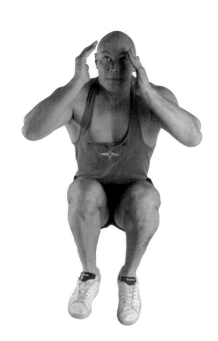

KNEES TO CHEST

Stand tall, back straight, with feet and knees together. Now, jump as high as you can bringing both knees up to the chest until your thighs are parallel to the ground. Throughout each repetition, face forwards and keep your back straight. Knees to chest exercises your calfs, quads, hamstrings, gluteus maximus (buttocks) and hip flexors.

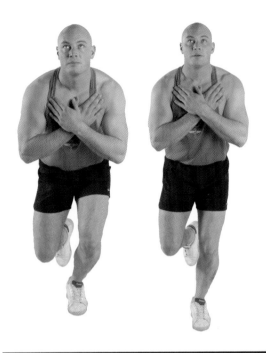

ONE-LEGGED SQUATS

Stand on your left leg with your arms across your chest. Now, bend your left leg until your right knee is as close to the floor as possible, hold for one second and extend your left leg. Do as many repetitions as you can, then repeat on your right leg.

WHOLE BODY EXERCISES

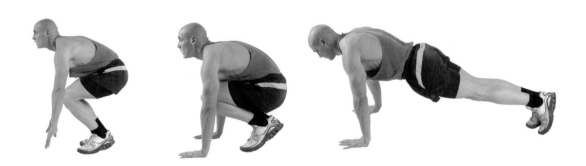

BURPEES

From a standing position, drop to the floor and assume a crouch position, then fully extend your legs backwards, thrust your legs back to the crouching position, stand up and repeat.

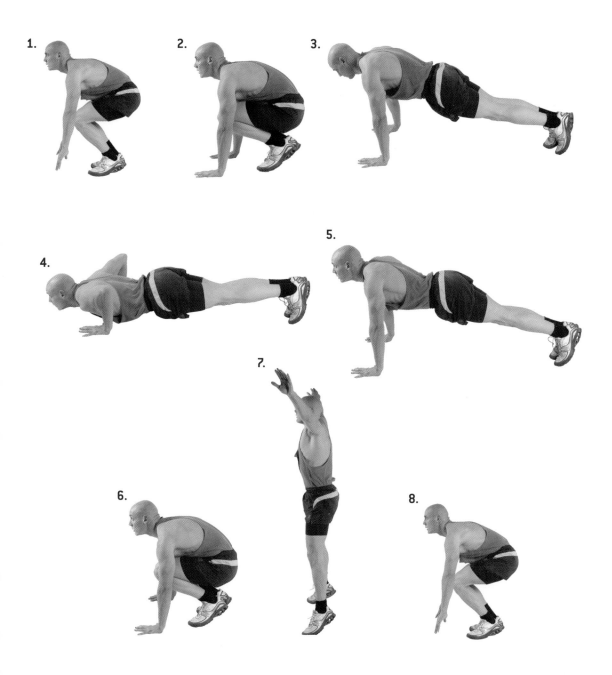

BASTARDS 🏋

Just as the title suggests, these are monster exercises! From a standing position, drop to a crouching position, thrust your legs backwards, complete one full press-up, jump your legs back to the crouching position, perform a star jump and then repeat.

TIPS

TIPS, HINTS AND EXPLANATIONS FOR ALL EXERCISE PROGRAMMES

REMEMBER: All training sessions should be started with a comprehensive warm-up and cool-down as described in Part 4.

COMPONENTS OF FITNESS

Endurance

Aerobic endurance is the term given to the capacity of your heart and lungs to send oxygen to your muscles in order to sustain a specific level of activity, e.g. running.

Muscular endurance refers to the capacity of a muscle, or muscle group, to perform repeated contractions against a resistance for an extended period of time, e.g. the ability to perform 500 press-ups without rest.

Strength

Strength relates to your body's capacity to exert force on physical objects using muscles. Weightlifting is a good example of strength training as the aim is to condition the muscle to maximize its power, and often its size. Strength often comes at the expense of peak aerobic performance because muscle bulk prevents the body from moving efficiently.

Speed

Speed can relate to either the time taken to transport the whole body over a distance, or to co-ordinate joint actions. Speed depends on the level of flexibility and must be developed in parallel with strength.

Flexibility

The ability of your joints to move through a full range of motions. Having flexibility in your muscles allows for more movement around the joints which improves endurance, strength and speed as well as making your body less susceptible to injury. Flexibility is developed through stretching exercises.

Cardiovascular Fitness (CV)

The term given to describe fitness exercises that develop heart and lung fitness along with the major muscle groups.

Interval Training

A series of repetitions of high intensity training interspersed with rest periods.

Hill Reps

An interval training session where a hill is used to increase the intensity of intervals rather than pace.

Active Rest

A rest period where the physical activity is continued, but at a lower intensity.

JUDGING CARDIOVASCULAR EXERCISE INTENSITY:

Training Zone	Spartan Method	Emperor Method
Moderate activity zone: 50–60% effort	You are able to talk	50–60% of maximum heart rate
Weight management zone: 60–70% effort	You can use short sentences only	60–70% of maximum heart rate
Aerobic zone: 70–80% effort	You can utter a few words at a time	70–80% of maximum heart rate
Anaerobic threshold zone: 80–90% effort	You are only able to say one word at a time	80–90% of maximum heart rate
Redline zone: 90–100% effort	There is no chance of you being able to talk	90–100% of maximum heart rate

- **Moderate activity zone:** Can feel pretty boring, burns more fat than carbohydrates.
- **Weight management zone:** Great for the heart, giving it the opportunity to work at its optimum level for a sustained period.
- **Aerobic zone:** The optimum zone to get fitter, faster and stronger.
- **Anaerobic threshold zone:** This training zone gives a training intensity where your body is just able to provide enough oxygen to power your muscles.
- **Redline zone:** This is the highest intensity training zone, which should not to be entered unless you are extremely fit.

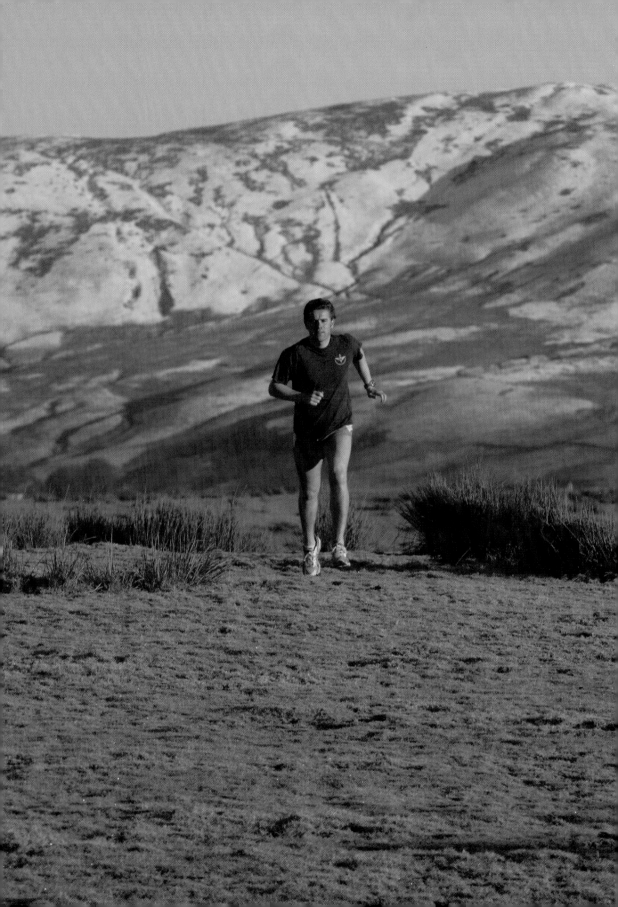

SPARTAN RECRUIT (BASIC LEVEL) PROGRAMME

	Day 1	Day 2	Day 3	Day 4	Notes
Week 1	Assessment: PARA Entry Test, see pages 38–40	Aerobic: 20min jog/walk @ 50%	Strength: 3x 10 press-ups (choice) 3x 10 dips (choice) 3x 10 sit-ups (choice) 3x 20sec core (choice) 3x 10 legs (choice)	Aerobic: 20min jog/walk @ 50%	Record results of assessment to compare at Weeks 4 and 8
Week 2	Strength: 3x 10 press-ups (choice) 3x 10 dips (choice) 3x 10 sit-ups (choice) 3x 20sec core (choice) 3x 10 legs (choice)	Aerobic: 25min jog/walk @ 50%	Strength: 3x 12 press-ups (choice) 3x 12 dips (choice) 3x 12 sit-ups (choice) 3x 25sec core (choice) 3x 12 legs (choice)	Aerobic: 25min jog/walk @ 50%	
Week 3	Aerobic: 25min jog/walk @ 60%	Strength: 3x 15 press-ups (choice) 3x 15 dips (choice) 3x 15 sit-ups (choice) 3x 30sec core (choice) 3x 15 legs (choice)	Aerobic: 30min jog/walk @ 50%	Strength: 3x 15 press-ups (choice) 3x 15 dips (choice) 3x 15 sit-ups (choice) 3x 30sec core (choice) 3x 15 legs (choice)	
Week 4	Strength: 3x 15 press-ups (choice) 3x 15 dips (choice) 3x 15 sit-ups (choice) 3x 30sec core (choice) 3x 15 legs (choice)	Aerobic: 30min jog/walk @ 50%	Strength: 3x 17 press-ups (choice) 3x 17 dips (choice) 3x 17 sit-ups (choice) 3x 40sec core (choice) 3x 17 legs (choice)	Assessment: PARA Entry Test, see pages 38–40	Compare scores to Day 1, Week 1 assessment

SPARTAN RECRUIT PROGRAMME (CONTINUED)

	Day 1	Day 2	Day 3	Day 4	Notes
Week 5	Aerobic: 30min jog @ 60% 2 hill reps @ 70%	Strength: 3x 17 press-ups (choice) 3x 17 dips (choice) 3x 17 sit-ups (choice) 3x 40sec core (choice) 3x 17 legs (choice)	Aerobic: 30min jog @ 60% 2 hill reps @ 70%	Strength: 3x 18 press-ups (choice) 3x 18 dips (choice) 3x 18 sit-ups (choice) 3x 45sec core (choice) 3x 18 legs (choice)	All interval sessions should be undertaken as an integral activity in the middle of your training session
Week 6	Strength: 3x 18 press-ups (choice) 3x 18 dips (choice) 3x 18 sit-ups (choice) 3x 45sec core (choice) 3x 18 legs (choice)	Aerobic: 30min jog @ 60% 4 hill reps @ 70%	Strength: 3x 20 press-ups (choice) 3x 20 dips (choice) 3x 20 sit-ups (choice) 3x 45sec core (choice) 3x 20 legs (choice)	Aerobic: 35min jog @ 60% 4 hill reps @ 70%	
Week 7	Aerobic: 35min jog @ 60% 6 hill reps @ 70%	Strength: 3x 20 press-up (choice) 3x 20 dips (choice) 3x 20 sit-ups (choice) 3x 45sec core (choice) 3x 20 legs (choice)	Aerobic: 45min jog @ 60%	Strength: 3x 20 press-ups (choice) 3x 20 dips (choice) 3x 20 sit-ups (choice) 3x 45sec core (choice) 3x 20 legs (choice)	
Week 8	Strength: 3x 22 press-ups (choice) 3x 22 dips (choice) 3x 22 sit-ups (choice) 3x 50sec core (choice) 3x 22 legs (choice)	Aerobic: 45min jog @ 60% 4 hill reps @ 70%	Strength: 3x 22 press-ups (choice) 3x 22 dips (choice) 3x 22 sit-ups (choice) 3x 50sec core (choice) 3x 22 legs (choice)	Assessment: PARA Entry Test, see page 38–40	Compare scores to Day 4, Week 4 assessment

SPARTAN SOLDIER (INTERMEDIATE LEVEL) PROGRAMME

	Day 1	Day 2	Day 3	Day 4	Notes
Week 1	Assessment: PARA Entry Test, see pages 38–40	Strength: 3x 20 press-ups (choice) 3x 20 dips (choice) 3x 20 sit-ups (choice) 3x 45sec core (choice) 3x 20 legs (choice)	Aerobic: 30min run @ 60% 5x 100m intervals @ 70% 100m recovery each	Aerobic / Strength: 35min run @ 60% 3x hill reps @ 70% 3x 15 press-ups (choice) 3x 15 sit-ups (choice) 3x 30sec core (choice)	Record results of assessment to compare at Weeks 4 and 8
Week 2	Aerobic: 20min run @ 60% 3x hill reps @ 70% Walk down recovery 3x 100m efforts @ 70% 100m recovery each	Strength: 3x 22 press-ups (choice) 3x 22 dips (choice) 3x 22 sit-ups (choice) 3x 45sec core (choice) 3x 22 legs (choice)	Aerobic: 40min jog @ 60% (undulating ground) 5x 30sec intervals @ 80%	Strength: 3x 22 press-ups (choice) 3x 22 dips (choice) 3x 22 sit-ups (choice) 3x 45sec core (choice) 3x 22 legs (choice)	
Week 3	Aerobic: 25min jog @ 60% (undulating ground) 10x 30 interval sprints	Strength: 3x 24 press-ups (choice) 3x 24 dips (choice) 3x 24 sit-ups (choice) 3x 50sec core (choice) 3x 24 legs (choice) 3x 5 pull-ups (choice)	Aerobic: 8x 200m @ 70% 200m recovery 8x 100m @ 70% 100m recovery	Strength: 3x 24 press-ups (choice) 3x 24 dips (choice) 3x 24 sit-ups (choice) 3x 50sec core (choice) 3x 24 legs (choice) 3x 5 pull-ups (choice)	All interval sessions should be undertaken as an integral activity in the middle of your training session
Week 4	Aerobic: Warm-up 50min run @ 60%	Strength: 3x 25 press-ups (choice) 3x 25 dips (choice) 3x 25 sit-ups (choice) 3x 50sec core (choice) 3x 25 legs (choice) 3x 6 pull-ups (choice)	Aerobic: 20min run @ 60% 6x 200m @ 70% 200m recovery 6x 100m @ 70% 100m recovery	Assessment: PARA Entry Test, see pages 38–40	Compare scores to Day 1, Week 1 assessment

SPARTAN SOLDIER PROGRAMME (CONTINUED)

	Day 1	Day 2	Day 3	Day 4	Notes
Week 5	Aerobic: 20min run @ 60% 5x 2min intervals @ 80% 4min recovery each	Strength: 3x 20 press-ups (choice) 3x 20 dips (choice) 3x 20 sit-ups (choice) 3x 45sec core (choice) 3x 20 legs (choice) 3x 5 pull-ups Select more difficult exercises than Weeks 1–4	Aerobic: 25min run @ 60% 8x 200m intervals @ 70% 200m recovery 8x 100m intervals @ 70% 100m recovery	Aerobic: 50min run @ 70%	All interval sessions should be undertaken as an integral activity in the middle of your training session
Week 6	Aerobic: 30min run @ 60% 5x 1min intervals @ 80% 2min recovery per rep	Strength: 3x 20 press-ups (choice) 3x 20 dips (choice) 3x 20 sit-ups (choice) 3x 45sec core (choice) 3x 20 legs (choice) 3x 5 pull-ups Select more difficult exercises than Weeks 1–4	Aerobic: 20min run @ 60% 8x 200m @ 80% 200m recovery per rep 8x 100m @ 80% 100m recovery per rep	Strength: 3x 22 press-ups (choice) 3x 22 dips (choice) 3x 22 sit-ups (choice) 3x 50sec core (choice) 3x 22 legs (choice) 3x 6 pull-ups Select more difficult exercises than Weeks 1–4	
Week 7	Aerobic: 50min run @ 70%	Strength: 3x 22 press-up (choice) 3x 22 dips (choice) 3x 22 sit-ups (choice) 3x 50sec core (choice) 3x 22 legs (choice) 3x 6 pull-ups Select more difficult exercises than Weeks 1–4	Aerobic: 60min run @ 60% (undulating ground) 8x 30 secs intervals @ 90%	Aerobic / Strength: 35min run @ 60% 3x hill reps @ 70% 3x 20 press-up (choice) 3x 20 sit-ups (choice) 3x 60sec core (choice) Select more difficult exercises than Weeks 1–4	
Week 8	Aerobic: 20min run @ 60% 5x hill reps @ 80% Walk down for recovery 5x 100m @ 80% 100m recovery per rep	Strength: 3x 24 press-ups (choice) 3x 24 dips (choice) 3x 24 sit-ups (choice) 3x 60sec core (choice) 3x 24 legs (choice) 3x 7 pull-ups Select more difficult exercises than Weeks 1–4	Aerobic: 40min run @ 70%	Assessment: PARA Entry Test, see pages 38–40	Compare scores to Day 4, Week 4 assessment.

SPARTAN PARATROOPER (HIGH LEVEL) PROGRAMME

	Day 1	Day 2	Day 3	Day 4	Notes
Week 1	Assessment: Five-Minute Test see pages 135–136 6-mile run best effort BMI Reach Test	Strength: 3x 20 press-ups (choice) 3x 20 dips (choice) 3x 20 sit-ups (choice) 3x 45sec core (choice) 3x 20 legs (choice) 3x 8 pull-ups (all at least soldier-level)	Aerobic: Warm-up 60min run (undulating ground) with 8x 30sec sprints en route 10min cool-down with stretching	Aerobic / Strength: 30min run @ 70% 3x hill reps @ 80% 3x 20 press-ups 3x 20 sit-ups 3x 60sec plank (all at least soldier-level)	Record results of assessment to compare at Weeks 4 and 8. All interval sessions should be undertaken as an integral activity in the middle of your training session
Week 2	Aerobic: 60min run @ 70%	Strength: 3x 20 press-ups (choice) 3x 20 dips (choice) 3x 20 sit-ups (choice) 3x 45sec core (choice) 3x 20 legs (choice) 3x 8 pull-ups (all at least soldier-level)	Aerobic: 35min run @ 60% 5x hill reps (200m) @ 80% Jog/walk down to recover	Strength: 3x 22 press-ups (choice) 3x 22 dips (choice) 3x 22 sit-ups (choice) 3x 60sec core (choice) 3x 22 legs (choice) 3x 10 pull-ups (all at least soldier-level)	
Week 3	Aerobic: 40min run @ 60% 5x hill reps (200m) @ 80% Jog/walk down to recover	Strength: 3x 22 press-ups (choice) 3x 22 dips (choice) 3x 22 sit-ups (choice) 3x 60sec core (choice) 3x 22 legs (choice) 3x 10 pull-ups (all at least soldier-level)	Aerobic: 30min run @ 70% 5x 100m @ 80% 100m recovery per rep	Aerobic / Strength: 40min run @ 70% 3x hill reps @ 80% 3x 22 press-ups 3x 22 sit-ups 3x 60sec plank (all at least soldier-level)	
Week 4	Aerobic: 20min run @ 70% 5x 100m hill reps @ 80% Walk down for recovery 5x 100m @ 80% 100m recovery per rep	Strength: 3x 25 press-ups (choice) 3x 25 dips (choice) 3x 25 sit-ups (choice) 3x 60sec core (choice) 3x 25 legs (choice) 3x 12 pull-ups (all at least soldier-level)	Aerobic: 45min run @ 60% 5x hill reps (200m) @ 80% Jog/walk down to recover	Assessment: Five-Minute Test 6-mile run best effort BMI Reach Test	Compare scores to Day 1, Week 1 assessment.

SPARTAN PARATROOPER PROGRAMME (CONTINUED)

	Day 1	Day 2	Day 3	Day 4	Notes
Week 5	Aerobic: 90min run @ 70%	Strength: 4x 20 press-ups (choice) 4x 20 dips (choice) 4x 20 sit-ups (choice) 4x 45sec core (choice) 4x 20 legs (choice) 4x 8 pull-ups (all at least soldier-level)	Aerobic: 20min run @ 70% 6x 200m @ 80% 200m recovery 6x 100m @ 80% 100m recovery	Aerobic / Strength: 60min run @ 70% 3x hill reps @ 80% 3x 25 press-ups 3x 25 sit-ups 3x 60sec plank (all at least soldier-level)	All interval sessions should be undertaken as an integral activity in the middle of your training session
Week 6	Aerobic: 15min run @ 60% with 8x 90sec sprints at 80% en route 3min active recovery per rep	Strength: 4x 22 press-ups (choice) 4x 22 dips (choice) 4x 22 sit-ups (choice) 4x 60sec core (choice) 4x 22 legs (choice) 4x 10 pull-ups (all at least soldier-level)	Aerobic: 15min run @ 60% with 5x 60sec sprints at 90% en route 3min active recovery per rep	Strength: 4x 22 press-ups (choice) 4x 22 dips (choice) 4x 22 sit-ups (choice) 4x 60sec core (choice) 4x 22 legs (choice) 4x 10 pull-ups (all at least soldier-level)	
Week 7	Aerobic: 40min run @ 70% (undulating ground) with 8x 30sec sprints @ 90% en route	Strength: 4x 24 press-ups (choice) 4x 24 dips (choice) 4x 24 sit-ups (choice) 4x 70sec core (choice) 4x 24 legs (choice) 4x 12 pull-ups (all at least soldier-level)	Aerobic: 80min run @ 70% (undulating ground)	Aerobic / Strength: 60min run @ 70% 4x hill reps @ 80% 4x 25 press-ups 4x 25 sit-ups 4x 60sec plank (all at least soldier-level)	
Week 8	Aerobic: 20min run @ 70% 5x 150m hill reps @ 80% Walk down for recovery 5x 100m sprints @ 90% 100m recovery per rep	Strength: 4x 24 press-ups (choice) 4x 24 dips (choice) 4x 24 sit-ups (choice) 4x 70sec core (choice) 4x 24 legs (choice) 4x 12 pull-ups (all at least soldier-level)	Aerobic: 30min run @ 70% 5x 1min sprints @ 90% 2min recovery per rep	Assessment: Five-Minute Test 10-mile run best effort BMI Reach Test	Separate run and other tests by at least an hour

The Five-Minute Test

For those who turn their nose up at the PARA Entrance Test as an assessment, because it's not tough enough – I'm not convinced. Anything best effort by definition should see you working at your performance threshold and it's a useful gauge of all-round fitness. However, for those who want something a bit special, replace the 1½-mile run with a six- or ten-mile run instead and use the Five-Minute Test instead of the press-ups, pull-ups and sit-ups. Don't be fooled by its simplicity – done properly it can feel just as tough as a VO2 Max test!

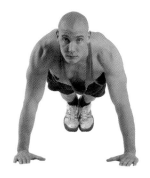

The Five-Minute Test, while an unofficial assessment, is widely used throughout the PARAS to assess fitness. I have used it on every operational tour I've deployed on, both as a test and a fitness session in itself; it makes for a very long five minutes! The mix and duration and the brief rest between each exercise makes it an awesome assessment of both muscular endurance and cardiovascular fitness. The primitive

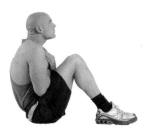

PERFORMANCE STANDARDS				
Cardiovascular Fitness Activity	Basic	Recruit	Soldier	Paratrooper
Running				
1½ miles	12.31–18min	10.30–12.30min	8.00–10.31min	Under 8min
6 miles	51–75min	43–50.59min	35–42.59min	Under 35min
10 miles	87–125min	75–87min	60–75min	Under 60min
Muscular Endurance	Combined Total Exercises			
Five-Minute Test • Press-ups (1min) • Sit-ups (1min) • Star jumps (1min) • Squat thrusts (1min) • Burpees (1min) • 10sec rest between each exercise	0–99	100–199	200–264	Over 265

nature of the assessment, combined with the lack of any need for space or specialized equipment, makes it one of my favourite fitness challenges. There is no requirement to do the exercises in a particular order, but I recommend using the following order to maximize your total: press-ups, sit-ups, squat thrusts, star jumps and finally burpees. When attempting this test for the first time, I would recommend doing a rehearsal a couple of days before, to get your transition between exercises right and prepare yourself mentally.

By now you should have found a number of running routes of varying lengths. In order to maximize your chances of achieving a good time, you will need a route that has as few obstacles as possible, which ideally crosses no major roads and is well away from vehicle or pedestrian congestion. Depending on how your fitness has progressed try and increase your run to six or ten miles and use the table on page 135 to measure your progress.

DEPLOYMENT IN AFGHANISTAN

Fitness as escapism and stress relief

On my numerous operational deployments with the PARAS, I have witnessed the full spectrum of fitness facilities. In the immediate aftermath of the terrorist attacks on the Twin Towers in 2001, I was one of the first soldiers to enter Kabul. My platoon, 10 Platoon, D Company, 2 PARA, were a hardy band of men, with a mutual respect and trust for one another built on demanding training and facing a common adversity. At the time we were the holders of the Bruneval Cup, a competition fiercely fought out to identify 2 PARA's best platoon. We had won the title largely due to our supreme fitness, which was exceptional even by PARA standards. This fitness had been hard to attain and we were all equally committed to preserving it during our four-month, short-notice Afghan deployment.

From our quarters in a bombed-out former Russian barracks, I observed the sort of ingenuity and resourcefulness that is the trademark of airborne soldiers. Using a selection of equipment that was either bought from the local bazaar, or

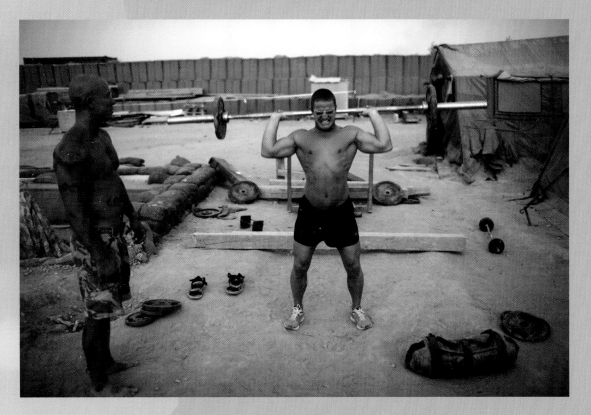

borrowed and misused from the quartermasters' department, we created a gym within a week of arriving. In the months that followed, our improvised gym not only kept us fit for our demanding patrol programme but provided some escapism from the intense Taliban insurgency we were fighting against. The hours we spent in our makeshift gym were social occasions and a daily ritual. Looking back, it was as much about relieving the stress of the day through reciprocal banter as it was about coming together to beat yesterday's performance and beast one another.

On my most recent tour in Afghanistan, I noticed that along with the rest of the infrastructure, military gyms have come on a long way, the norm now being aircraft hangars filled with state-of-the-art fitness equipment. However, their purpose remains the same – keeping soldiers mentally and physically fit to fight tomorrow's challenges.

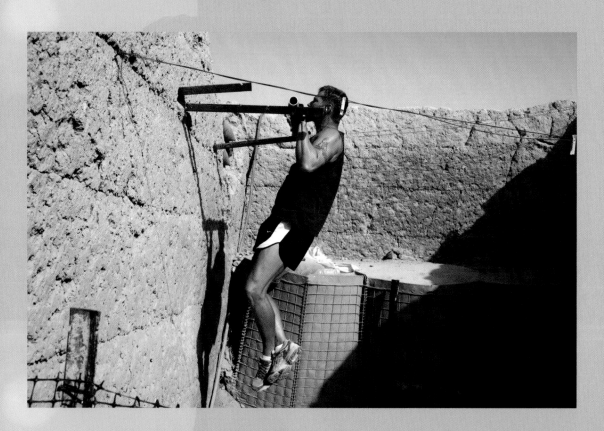

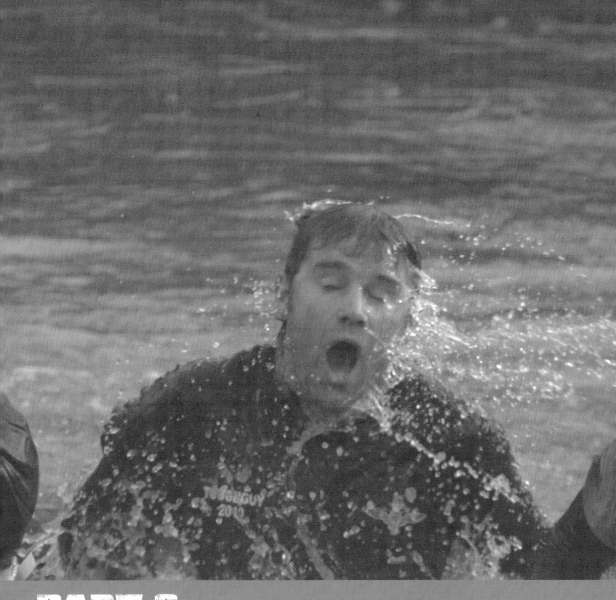

PART 6
THE P COMPANY EMPEROR
PROGRAMME (WITH FRILLS)

'Luxury must be comfortable, otherwise it is not luxury'
Coco Chanel

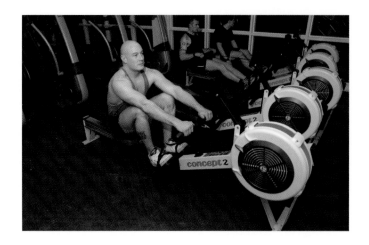

During my 12 years in the Parachute Regiment, I've yet to come across a paratrooper who enjoys being cold and wet, and our new recruits seem to like it the least. The Spartan approach we use to turn civilians into paratroopers is as much about developing hardiness and resilience in potential PARAS as it is about physical fitness. In PARA recruits, a lack of faith or commitment to their training syllabus results in them failing to achieve both their goal and their potential.

For many reading this book, the programme inspired by PARA basic training in Part 5 would soon become monotonous and ultimately be abandoned. For potential PARA recruits, the pace and path of the transition from Clark Kent to Superman is dictated to them. You, however, have choice! Choice to purchase this book – a good start – choice to embark on a new fitness training regime, choice over how hard, when and how you train and choice to stick at it.

In this part, you will develop the knowledge and skills required to create a programme that achieves your fitness goals in a manner that is supported by your lifestyle and interests. But first a word of caution. While it is possible to steer a course away from monotony and bad weather, persistence and hard work lie at the heart of every successful exercise programme.

In the previous chapter, my focus was the destination – getting you paratrooper-fit, using nothing more than a pair of trainers, a watch, and blood, sweat and tears. I would describe this chapter as Part 5's equivalent of flying First Class; while the destination is the same and there may still be some turbulence along the way, the journey is much more pleasant.

Fitness programmes alone won't get you fit, but your commitment to the right fitness programme will. Sustainability is the key. Before

I explain some of the various fun, interesting and fitness-enhancing activities you can use to get paratrooper-fit and maintain your commitment in the process, I must emphasize that choice comes with a responsibility. This responsibility is to realistically commit to a goal and a method of achieving it that not only fits with your lifestyle, but is supported by the time and money at your disposal and the environment in which you live. So, assuming you are comfortable with this responsibility, let's introduce some luxury and make your journey to paratrooper fitness more akin to Concorde than Colditz.

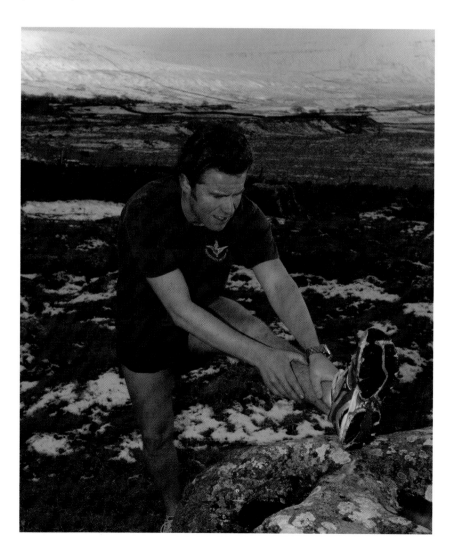

The Gym

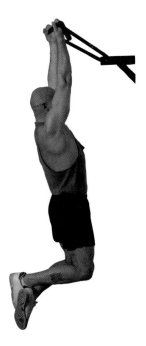

As was illustrated in the account of 10 Platoon's tour in Afghanistan in 2001, gyms are not only brilliant places to hone your fitness, but are also social settings where you can meet up with friends. After all, daily stress is not solely the preserve of Afghanistan, and physical fitness is a currency whose value extends far beyond war zones. In this section, we will explore some criteria for assessing whether training in a gym is right for you and, if it is, how to select the right gym and get the most from it. However, as with every section of this book, the starting point is asking yourself what you want from a gym, and when you intend to use it. Once you have a clear answer to these questions there are three important areas of any potential gym that should be evaluated.

SERVICE

Gyms provide a service and it is important to find one that is goal-enhancing and configured for your convenience. When I commanded the PARA recce platoon, we had a saying: 'time spent on reconnaissance is never wasted'. I believe this is equally true when scoping out gyms. During your recce here are some things to look for:

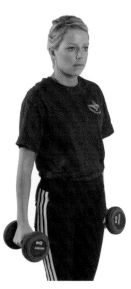

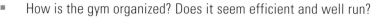

- How is the gym organized? Does it seem efficient and well run?
- What type of equipment does it have? What state is it in and how does it compare to what you're looking for?
- Do the staff and other members make you feel comfortable?
- What do the other members say about the staff?
- What qualifications do the staff have and what classes do they offer?
- A good test is asking what happens if you forget your membership card – if their answer is that they deny you access then it is probably best to cut short your visit.

COST

Gym memberships are priced to attract people to join for an extended period (normally a year) because statistically most clients won't use the gym much after mid-January. Work out what it is you want from a gym, if it is merely weights then the jacuzzi, aerobics classes, outdoor swimming pool and other facilities are a waste of your membership fees. You will pay a premium for prime-time usage, but if you were planning to only use the gym at off-peak times, you may be able to negotiate a cheaper membership that only includes the relevant time window.

CONVENIENCE

Above all else, your gym needs to fit around your lifestyle. Being located close to work, home, or at least en-route is a critical success factor. What is the traffic and parking like at the times when you'll be visiting it? When is it open and how busy is it when you intend to do most of your training? Are towels and lockers provided? Can you leave your kit there? Make sure you go to the gym knowing exactly what you want from it and when you intend to use it, and don't be seduced by the honey trap of a good-looking sales person playing to your ego. The gym either has what you need or it doesn't. If possible, try before you buy and do a full dress rehearsal at exactly the time you intend to train. Look for potential pitfalls – if you're struggling to make it fit, it probably doesn't.

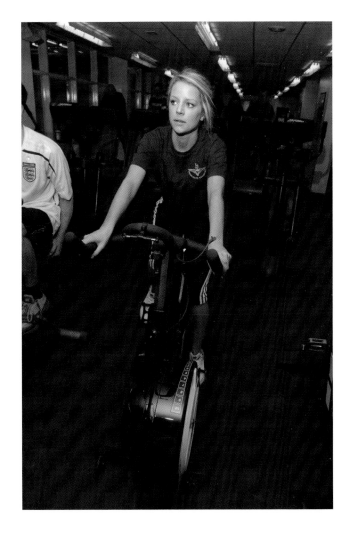

Personal Trainers

If you can afford a personal trainer there is no doubt that a good one will seriously enhance the effectiveness of your exercise programme. All personal trainers will be REPS 3 qualified, which to an extent ensures that they know what they are talking about.

The relationship you have with your personal trainer is not just one of the critical success factors in your training, but possibly the most important one. Central to the relationship is mutual trust, confidentiality, empathy and acceptance of your goals and ability. Equally important is your personal trainer's credibility and confidence (but not ego), which will enhance your confidence in them. For me, the most important factor is role modelling – your personal trainer needs to practice what they preach and have the experience of having trained hard for a specific goal over an extended period, otherwise how else can they understand what you will be going through? After that, the most important factor is getting a feeling for their ability to blend authentic support with challenge in order to aid your development. If you are thinking of employing a personal trainer, I would suggest asking them a few penetrating questions about their training first and then go with your gut instinct. Also, don't be afraid to ask for a free trial session. However, most personal trainers are self-employed and pay a ground rent for working in a gym, so they might not be able to afford to do this as it would literally be costing them money.

Rowing

Rowing is a good all-round exercise, which develops your strength, speed and endurance. This blend of fitness training makes rowing suitable for every fitness programme, regardless of your age or fitness level. Below are but a few of the many benefits derived from rowing as an exercise:

- It provides a superb aerobic workout.
- In terms of calorie-burning, it is up there at the top with running and cycling (see page 55).
- It exercises every major muscle group.
- The monitor provides accurate feedback on session progress, and overall training progress.
- It is a time-efficient form of exercise and an excellent stress-reliever.
- It is weight-supporting and non-jarring and so is ideal for rehabilitative exercise.
- It can be a very effective fat-burning and weight-loss exercise.
- It is suitable for people of all ages.

I have been integrating rowing into my personal exercise regime for nearly 15 years. What I really like about it, even more than the full body workout it delivers, is the immediate performance feedback you get from the machine's display. However, technique is the most important factor when using the rowing machine, and more people get it wrong than right. If you get your technique right, you'll be efficient, produce better scores/results and avoid potential injuries. I can't recommend this machine enough.

ROWING TECHNIQUE

Sit on the rower and lean back slightly, legs flat, handle drawn to the body with your forearms horizontal. To start the motion your arms

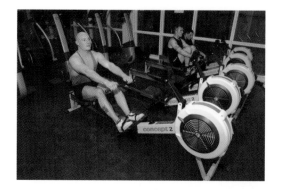
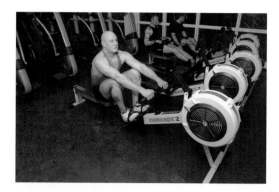
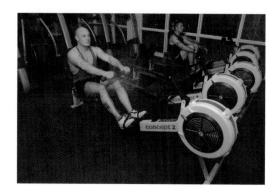
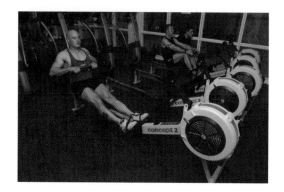

should be relaxed and extended fully. The body rocks forwards from the hips. Once your arms have fully extended and the body is rocked forward, slide forwards maintaining arm and body position. Your shins should now be vertical, with your body pressed up to your legs. From here the legs push down and the body begins to lever back. The legs continue to push as the body levers back; throughout, ensure your arms remain straight. The arms draw the handle past the knees and then strongly up to the body, returning to the finish position as if you're elbowing someone behind you. You are now ready to take the next stroke.

Cycling

After running and rowing, cycling is my favourite fitness activity and one of the best forms of exercise available. Both mountain and road bikes can be purchased relatively cheaply. Perhaps the best reason to use a bike is that you are able to exercise at a high intensity without any significant jarring on your joints. For me, one of the real appeals of cycling is the chance to see a wider area during a training period than you ever could running.

As an exercise, cycling offers numerous benefits. The heart and legs take on most of the work, but the stomach and arms also get a great workout from cycling. Cycling at a high intensity has huge calorie-burning potential, metamorphosing fat into lean muscle far quicker than most other exercises. Unless you choose to take up cycling on a static exercise bike, you will need some equipment to get started.

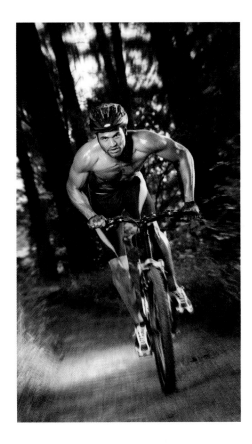

ESSENTIALS
You will need all of the following:

- A bike.
- A helmet.
- Padded shorts.

ADDED EXTRAS
The following won't do the work for you, but they will enhance your cycling experience:

- Cycling shoes, which clip into specially designed pedals – these make the energy transfer much more efficient during each pedal rotation.

- An odometer – this will give you instant feedback on your performance including:
  - Your speed.
  - How far you have travelled.
  - The cadence of your pedalling.
  - A link to your heart rate monitor.
- A combined GPS, heart-rate monitor and odometer computer system – this provides the most accurate feedback on your session.

Cycle training should be approached in much the same way as running training, with the following key stages:

STEADY STATE

This is when you cycle at an even pace throughout your training session. As soon as you're able to sustain a moderate cycle for about half an hour you are ready to take on something more advanced.

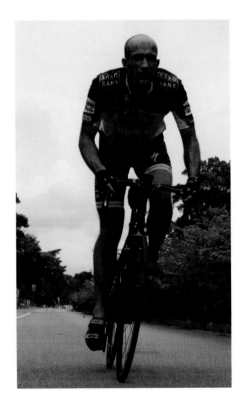

INTERVAL TRAINING

This is training at a specific intensity for a sustained period, followed by a rest, followed by repeating this process a number of times.

FARTLEK TRAINING

Like any other Fartlek training, this is when you vary your speed at different stages of a cycle ride, with set periods of faster, slower and sometimes intermediate-speed riding.

THRESHOLD SESSIONS

This is cycling at your threshold for a continuous period.

RECOVERY RIDES

A recovery ride is designed to allow the body to get rid of waste products from previous sessions.

Swimming

While swimming is not as efficient at burning calories as running, cycling or rowing, it remains an excellent activity which has next to no impact on your joints. It is the ideal training session for anyone who is either pregnant, overweight or recovering from a minor injury. Unfortunately, swimming is not something which can be learnt from a book and the best way to hone your technique is by consulting a specialist coach or joining a local club. Swimming training should be approached like any other individual endurance activity. To get the best results a combination of steady state, interval, Fartlek, threshold and recovery sessions should be undertaken.

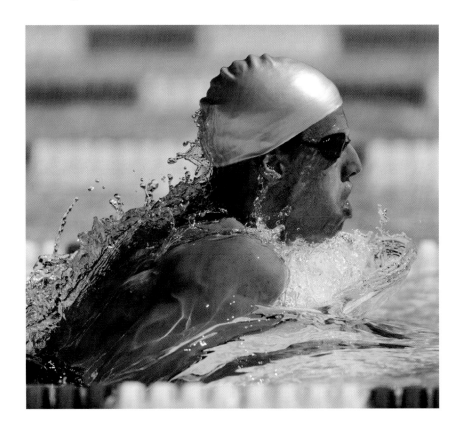

Other activities: Hill walking, Sports and Leisure activities

As I stated right at the beginning of this book, the secret to success in your fitness programme is finding activities that you enjoy, which deliver the training value you need for a particular session. If you manage to do this then it will be all the more likely that you will stick to your programme and ultimately achieve your goal. As a general rule, sports and leisure activities fall into one of three activities, though most overlap:

- Aerobic activity sports (e.g. hillwalking, aerobics classes, spinning classes, etc).
- Burst activity sports (e.g. competitive sports such as football, rugby, tennis, etc).
- Endurance sports (e.g. long-distance running/cycling, cross-country skiing, etc).

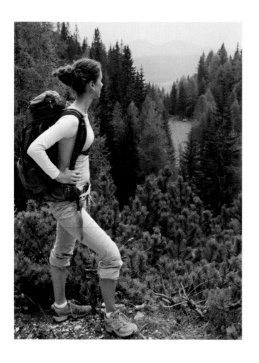

All of these can be great sessions to integrate into a fitness programme, particularly if you associate them with fun rather than viewing them as something to be endured in order to achieve a wider goal. I would urge you to look for as many opportunities as possible to do these types of activities in your training programme and there is nothing to stop you from bolting on some additional exercise to complement a session, if you think it appropriate. Whether your goal is performance- or health-based, the trick is to compare your choice of activities with what you seek to get from your training session – a good point of reference is probably the calorie-burning calculator on page 55; which allows you to compare the effects of different activities.

Weights

Regardless of how far you run or how much you circuit train, your muscles will be contracting against the same amount of resistance. This means that although you will get progressively fitter, your strength will start to plateau. As you now know, improvements come by forcing your body to adapt by overloading it with specific exercises. Weight training is widely recognised as the best progressive form of resistance training to build strength and muscle tone. First a word of caution, though: this section is meant as a general insight into weight training, and the training session is designed to complement a wider programme, not to turn you into Mr Universe. For that you need a much more specific programme, not to mention a meticulously planned diet. The focus here is increasing strength and muscular endurance. Before we commence here are some general principles.

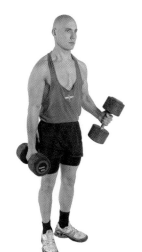

DIFFERENT GOALS OF WEIGHT TRAINING

- Strength endurance: This requires high repetitions (15-plus) with light loading (30–50% of your maximum for one repetition).
- Size and strength: This requires a medium to high number of repetitions (8–12) with medium to heavy loading (70–80%-plus of your maximum for one repetition).
- Power: This requires a medium number of repetitions (6–10) with medium to heavy loading (70–80% of your maximum for one repetition).
- Maximum strength: This requires a low number of repetitions (1–5) with heavy loads (80–100% of your maximum for one repetition).

Clearly, in order to progress you need to continually re-evaluate what your maximum for one repetition is, in order to increase the weights as you get stronger.

REST BETWEEN SETS (GROUPS OF REPETITIONS)

The aim of the recovery period is to allow your muscles to recover before the next set. Several factors influence the recovery period, including:

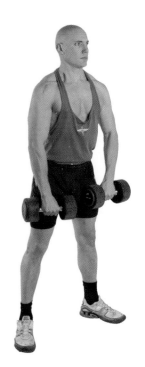

- The type of strength you are developing.
- The load used during the exercise.
- The number of muscle groups used during the exercise.
- Your condition.
- Your weight.

As a rule allow 1–2 minutes between each set. However, rather than squandering this time, do super sets. This is when you exercise different muscle groups back to back, thus each exercise provides the recovery time for the previous one.

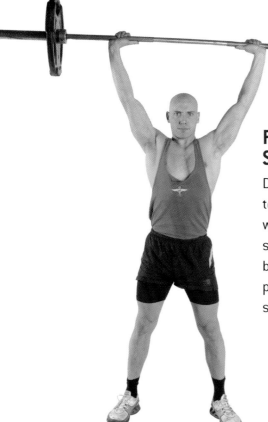

REST INTERVAL BETWEEN SESSIONS

Depending on your conditioning, it may be possible to train every 24 hours. However, as we are dealing with general weight training, rather than targeting specific muscle groups for a complete session, it is best to allow at least 48 hours for recovery – but be prepared for this not to be enough when you are starting off. Listen to your body.

WEIGHTLIFTING EXERCISES FOR YOUR SHOULDERS

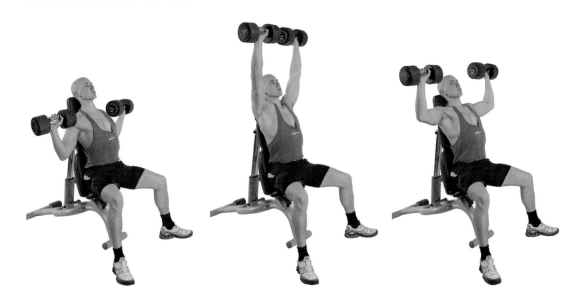

SHOULDER PRESS

Hold the dumb-bells at shoulder height, with your palms facing up. Keeping your back straight, raise the dumb-bells under control until your arms are fully extended, then gently lower.

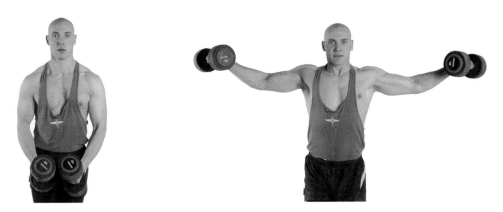

LATERAL SHOULDER RAISES

Stand with your legs shoulder-width apart and hold the dumb-bells with your palms facing inwards. With straight wrists and a slight bend at the elbow, raise your hands until they are in line with your shoulders, then return under control to your start position.

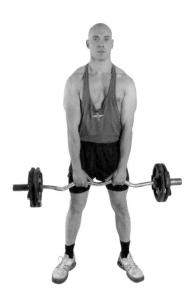 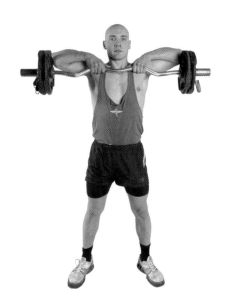

UPRIGHT ROW

Holding a barbell in front of you, with your palms facing down and your knuckles forwards, raise your arms until your elbows are higher than your shoulders before lowering under control.

WEIGHTLIFTING EXERCISES FOR YOUR ARMS

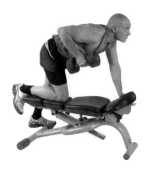 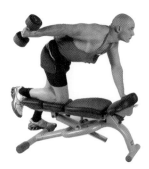

TRICEP KICK-BACK

Keep your back straight and parallel with the floor while resting your right knee and left arm on a weights bench. Hold the dumb-bell in your right arm with your palm facing in, next to your chest. Now, keeping your arm static above the elbow, extend your right arm backwards until it is parallel with your back, before gradually returning the weight to its starting position.

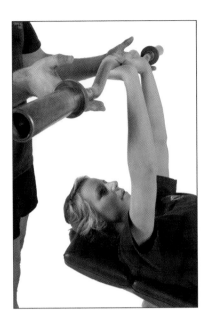

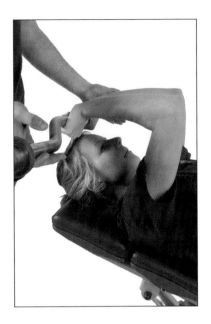

BARBELL PULL-OVER

Lying on your back, hold the barbell with your palms facing up and your elbows uppermost. Now, keeping your arms above your elbows static, bend your elbow until the weight is about an inch from your forehead, before returning to its start position under control. Do with assistance at first.

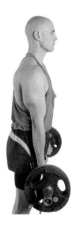

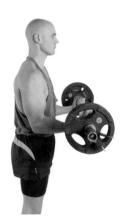

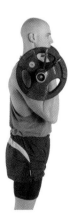

BARBELL CURLS

Hold the barbell with your palms up. Now, keeping your back straight, pivot your arms at the elbow to lift the weight until it is just above your shoulders, before lowering under control. By bringing your grip closer together, this exercise can also target your chest.

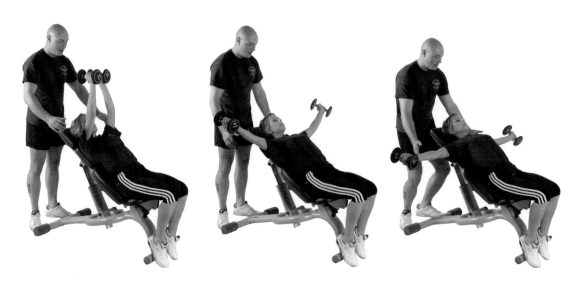

DUMB-BELL FLYS

Lying on your back on a bench, extend your arms in front of you and grip the dumb-bells with your palms facing in. With a slight bend in your elbow, lower your arms until the weights are in line with your chest, before raising your arms to their start position.

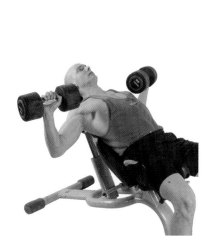

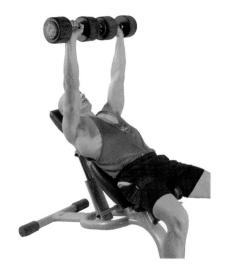

DUMB-BELL BENCH PRESS

Lie on a bench with your feet flat on the floor. Hold the dumb-bells with your palms facing inwards close to your chest. Now, raise your arms in front of you until they are fully extended, then return them to their starting position under control.

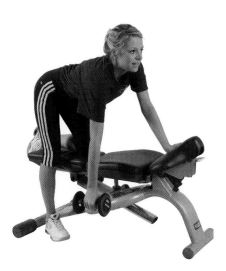 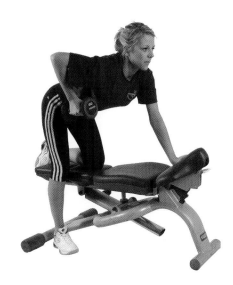

SINGLE DUMB-BELL ROW

Kneel on a bench with your left knee, supporting yourself with your left arm. Now holding the dumb-bell palm-down with your arm fully extended, lift it up until it is parallel with your chest before returning it to the start position under control. Repeat on the opposite side.

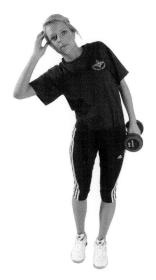 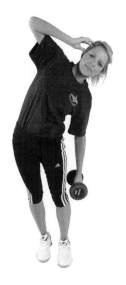

SIDE BEND

Hold a dumb-bell in your left hand with your legs slightly apart. Now reach down by your left leg, making sure you don't tilt either forwards or backwards. Reach as far down as is comfortable, before returning to the upright position. Repeat the exercise on your right side.

EMPEROR RECRUIT (BASIC LEVEL) PROGRAMME

	Day 1	Day 2	Day 3	Day 4	Notes
Week 1	Assessment: PARA Entry Test, see pages 38–40	Aerobic: 20min CV @ 50% or 30min competitive sport or 30min gym class	Strength: Weights 3x 8 @ 60% shoulders 3x 8 @ 60% triceps 3x 8 @ 60% barbell curl 3x 8 @ 60% chest 3x 8 @ 60% side bend 3x 20sec core (choice) 3x 10 leg circuit ex (choice)	Aerobic: 20min CV @ 50% or 30min competitive sport or 30min gym class	Record results of assessment to compare at Weeks 4 and 8 / All interval sessions should be undertaken as an integral activity in the middle of your training session
Week 2	Strength: 3x 10 press-ups (choice) 3x 10 dips (choice) 3x 10 sit-ups (choice) 3x 20sec core (choice) 3x 10 legs (choice)	Aerobic: 25min CV @ 50% or 25min competitive sport or 25min gym class	Strength: Weights 3x 9 @ 60% shoulders 3x 9 @ 60% triceps 3x 9 @ 60% barbell curl 3x 9 @ 60% chest 3x 9 @ 60% side bend 3x 30sec core (choice) 3x 15 leg circuit ex (choice)	Aerobic: 25min CV @ 50% or 30min competitive sport or 30min gym class	
Week 3	Aerobic: 25min CV @ 50% or 30min competitive sport or 30min gym class	Strength: 3x 15 press-ups (choice) 3x 15 dips (choice) 3x 15 sit-ups (choice) 3x 30sec core (choice) 3x 15 legs (choice)	Aerobic: 30min CV @ 50% or 30min competitive sport or 30min gym class	Strength: Weights 3x 10 @ 60% shoulders 3x 10 @ 60% triceps 3x 10 @ 60% barbell curl 3x 10 @ 60% chest 3x 10 @ 60% side bend 3x 30sec core (choice) 3x 15 leg circuit ex (choice)	
Week 4	Strength: 3x 15 press-ups (choice) 3x 15 dips (choice) 3x 15 sit-ups (choice) 3x 30sec core (choice) 3x 15 legs (choice)	Aerobic: 30min CV @ 50% or 30min competitive sport or 30min gym class	Strength: Weights 3x 11 @ 60% shoulders 3x 11 @ 60% triceps 3x 11 @ 60% barbell curl 3x 11 @ 60% chest 3x 11 @ 60% side bend 3x 30sec core (choice) 3x 15 leg circuit ex (choice)	Assessment: PARA Entry Test, see page 38–40	Compare scores to Day 1, Week 1 assessment

EMPEROR RECRUIT PROGRAMME (CONTINUED)

	Day 1	Day 2	Day 3	Day 4	Notes
Week 5	Aerobic: 35min CV @ 50% or 45min competitive sport or 45min gym class	Strength: 3x 17 press-ups (choice) 3x 17 dips (choice) 3x 17 sit-ups (choice) 3x 40sec core (choice) 3x 17 legs (choice)	Aerobic: 35min CV @ 50% or 45min competitive sport or 45min gym class	Strength: Weights 3x 12 @ 60% shoulders 3x 12 @ 60% triceps 3x 12 @ 60% barbell curl 3x 12 @ 60% chest 3x 12 @ 60% side bend 3x 40sec core (choice) 3x 17 leg circuit ex (choice)	All interval sessions should be undertaken as an integral activity in the middle of your training session
Week 6	Strength: 3x 18 press-ups (choice) 3x 18 dips (choice) 3x 18 sit-ups (choice) 3x 45sec core (choice) 3x 18 legs (choice)	Aerobic: 30min CV @ 60% 2 intervals @ 70% or 45min competitive sport or 45min gym class	Strength: Weights 3x 10 @ 70% shoulders 3x 10 @ 70% triceps 3x 10 @ 70% barbell curl 3x 10 @ 70% chest 3x 10 @ 70% side bend 3x 45sec core (choice) 3x 17 leg circuit ex (choice)	Aerobic: 30min CV @ 60% 4 intervals @ 70% or 45min competitive sport or 45min gym class	
Week 7	Aerobic: 30min CV @ 60% 6 intervals @ 70% or 60min competitive sport or 60min gym class	Strength: 3x 20 press-ups (choice) 3x 20 dips (choice) 3x 20 sit-ups (choice) 3x 45sec core(choice) 3x 20 legs (choice)	Aerobic: 45min CV @ 60% or 60min competitive sport or 60min gym class	Strength: Weights 3x 11 @ 70% shoulders 3x 11 @ 70% triceps 3x 11 @ 70% barbell curl 3x 11 @ 70% chest 3x 11 @ 70% side bend 3x 45sec core (choice) 3x 18 leg circuit ex (choice)	
Week 8	Strength: 3x 22 press-ups (choice) 3x 22 dips (choice) 3x 22 sit-ups (choice) 3x 50sec core (choice) 3x 22 legs (choice)	Aerobic: 45min CV @ 60% or 60min competitive sport or 60min gym class	Strength: Weights 3x 12 @ 70% shoulders 3x 12 @ 70% triceps 3x 12 @ 70% barbell curl 3x 12 @ 70% chest 3x 12 @ 70% side bend 3x 45sec core (choice) 3x 18 leg circuit ex (choice)	Assessment: PARA Entry Test, see pages 38–40	Compare scores to Day 4, Week 4 assessment

EMPEROR SOLDIER (INTERMEDIATE LEVEL) PROGRAMME

	Day 1	Day 2	Day 3	Day 4	Notes
Week 1	Assessment: PARA Entry Test pages 38–40	Strength: 3x 20 press-ups (choice) 3x 20 dips (choice) 3x 20 sit-ups (choice) 3x 45sec core (choice) 3x 20 legs (choice)	Aerobic: 30min CV @ 60% 5x 1min intervals @ 70% 1min recovery each or 60min competitive sport	Aerobic / Strength: 30min CV @ 60% 5x 1min intervals @ 70% 1min recovery each 3x 15 press-ups (choice) 3x 15 sit-ups (choice) 3x 30 sec core (choice)	Record results of assessment to compare at Weeks 4 and 8 All interval sessions should be undertaken as an integral activity in the middle of your training session
Week 2	Aerobic: 30min CV @ 60% 5x 1min intervals @ 70% 1min recovery each or 60min competitive sport	Strength: Weights 3x 12 @ 70% shoulders 3x 12 @ 70% triceps 3x 12 @ 70% barbell curl 3x 12 @ 70% chest 3x 12 @ 70% side bend 3x 45sec core (choice) 3x 18 leg circuit ex (choice)	Aerobic: 40min CV @ 60% 5x 30sec intervals @ 70% or 60min of competitive sport	Strength: 3x 22 press-ups (choice) 3x 22 dips (choice) 3x 22 sit-ups (choice) 3x 45sec core (choice) 3x 22 legs (choice)	
Week 3	Aerobic: 25min CV @ 60% 10x 30sec intervals	Strength: 3x 24 press-ups (choice) 3x 24 dips (choice) 3x 24 sit-ups (choice) 3x 50sec core (choice) 3x 24 legs (choice) 3x 5 pull-ups (choice)	Aerobic: 8x 1min @ 70% 1min recovery each 8x 30sec @ 70% 30sec recovery each	Strength: Weights 3x 12 @ 75% shoulders 3x 12 @ 75% triceps 3x 12 @ 75% barbell curl 3x 12 @ 75% chest 3x 12 @ 75% side bend 3x 50sec core (choice) 3x 18 leg circuit ex (choice)	
Week 4	Aerobic: 50min CV @ 60% or 60min competitive sport	Strength: Weights 3x 12 @ 80% shoulders 3x 12 @ 80% triceps 3x 12 @ 80% barbell curl 3x 12 @ 80% chest 3x 12 @ 80% side bend 3x 50sec core (choice) 3x 20 leg circuit ex (choice)	Aerobic: 20min CV @ 60% 6x 1min @ 70% 1min recovery each 6x 30sec @ 70% 30sec recovery each	Assessment: PARA Entry Test, see pages 38–40	Compare scores to Day 1, Week 1 assessment

EMPEROR SOLDIER PROGRAMME (CONTINUED)

	Day 1	Day 2	Day 3	Day 4	Notes
Week 5	Aerobic: 20min CV @ 60% 5x 2min intervals @ 80% 4min active recovery each or 75min of competitive sport	Strength: 3x 20 press-ups (choice) 3x 20 dips (choice) 3x 20 sit-ups (choice) 3x 45sec core (choice) 3x 20 legs (choice) 3x 5 pull-ups Select more difficult exercises than Weeks 1–4	Aerobic: 25min CV @ 60% 8x 1min intervals @ 70% 1min recovery each 8x 30sec intervals @ 70% 30sec recovery each	Strength: Weights 3x 12 @ 80% shoulders 3x 12 @ 80% triceps 3x 12 @ 80% barbell curl 3x 12 @ 80% chest 3x 12 @ 80% side bend 3x 50sec core (choice) 3x 20 leg circuit ex (choice)	All interval sessions should be undertaken as an integral activity in the middle of your training session
Week 6	Aerobic: 30mins CV @ 70% 5x 1min @ 80% 2min recovery per rep or 75min of competitive sport	Strength: 3x 20 press-ups (choice) 3x 20 dips (choice) 3x 22 sit-ups (choice) 3x 45sec core (choice) 3x 20 legs (choice) 3x 5 pull-ups Select more difficult exercises than Weeks 1–4	Aerobic: 20min CV @ 60% 8x 1min interval @ 80% 1min recovery per rep 8x 30sec interval @ 80% 30sec recovery per rep	Strength: Weights 3x 14 @ 80% shoulders 3x 14 @ 80% triceps 3x 14 @ 80% barbell curl 3x 14 @ 80% chest 3x 14 @ 80% side bend 3x 60sec core (choice) 3x 22 leg circuit ex (choice)	
Week 7	Aerobic: 50min CV @ 70% or 75min competitive sport	Strength: 3x 22 press-ups (choice) 3x 22 dips (choice) 3x 22 sit-ups (choice) 3x 50sec core (choice) 3x 22 legs (choice) 3x 6 pull-ups Select more difficult exercises than Weeks 1–4	Aerobic: 60min CV @ 60% 8x 30 secs @ 90%	Strength: Weights 3x 14 @ 80% shoulders 3x 14 @ 80% triceps 3x 14 @ 80% barbell curl 3x 14 @ 80% chest 3x 14 @ 80% side bend 3x 60sec core (choice) 3x 22 leg circuit ex (choice)	
Week 8	Aerobic: 20min CV @ 60% 5x 90sec intervals @ 80% 60sec recovery per rep 5x 45sec @ 80% 30sec recovery per rep or 75min competitive sport	Strength: 3x 24 press-ups (choice) 3x 24 dips (choice) 3x 24 sit-ups (choice) 3x 60sec core (choice) 3x 24 legs (choice) 3x 7 pull-ups Select more difficult exercises than Weeks 1–4	Aerobic: 45min CV @ 70%	Assessment: PARA Entry Test, see pages 38–40	Compare scores to Day 4, Week 4 assessment

EMPEROR PARATROOPER (HIGH LEVEL) PROGRAMME

	Day 1	Day 2	Day 3	Day 4	Notes
Week 1	Assessment: Five-Minute Test Middle distance CV test (choice) BMI Reach Test	Strength: 3x 20 press-ups (choice) 3x 20 dips (choice) 3x 20 sit-ups (choice) 3x 45sec core (choice) 3x 20 legs (choice) 3x 8 pull-ups (all at least soldier-level)	Aerobic: 60min CV @ 70% 8x 30sec intervals @ 80% 30sec recovery per rep	Strength: Weights 3x 15 @ 80% shoulders 3x 15 @ 80% triceps 3x 15 @ 80% barbell curl 3x 15 @ 80% chest 3x 15 @ 80% side bend 3x 60sec core (choice) 3x 22 leg circuit ex (choice)	Record results of assessment to compare at Weeks 4 and 8 All interval sessions should be undertaken as an integral activity in the middle of your training session
Week 2	Aerobic: 60min CV @ 70% or 90min competitive sport	Strength: 3x 20 press-ups (choice) 3x 20 dips (choice) 3x 20 sit-ups (choice) 3x 45sec core (choice) 3x 20 legs (choice) 3x 8 pull-ups (all at least soldier-level)	Aerobic: 35min CV @ 60% 5x 90sec intervals @ 80% 60sec recovery per rep	Strength: Weights 3x 15 @ 80% shoulders 3x 15 @ 80% triceps 3x 15 @ 80% barbell curl 3x 15 @ 80% chest 3x 15 @ 80% side bend 3x 60sec core (choice) 3x 22 leg circuit ex (choice)	
Week 3	Aerobic: Run 40min run @ 60% 5x hill reps (200m) @ 80% Jog/walk down to recover	Strength: 3x 22 press-ups (choice) 3x 22 dips (choice) 3x 22 sit-ups (choice) 3x 60sec core (choice) 3x 22 legs (choice) 3x 10 pull-ups (all at least soldier-level)	Aerobic: 30min CV @ 70% 5x 1min interval @ 80% 1min recovery per rep or 90min competitive sport	Aerobic / Strength: 40min CV @ 70% 3x 90sec intervals @ 80% 3x 22 press-ups 3x 22 sit-ups 3x 60sec plank (all at least soldier-level)	
Week 4	Aerobic: Run 20min run @ 70% 5x 100m hill reps at 80% Walk down for recovery 5x 100m @ 80% 100m recovery per rep	Strength: Weights 3x 15 @ 80% shoulders 3x 15 @ 80% triceps 3x 15 @ 80% barbell curl 3x 15 @ 80% chest 3x 15 @ 80% side bend 3x 60sec core (choice) 3x 22 leg circuit ex (choice)	Aerobic: 45min CV @ 60% 5x 90sec intervals @ 80% 30sec recovery per rep	Assessment: Five-Minute Test Middle-distance CV test (choice) BMI Reach Test	Compare scores to Day 1, Week 1 assessment

EMPEROR PARATROOPER PROGRAMME (CONTINUED)

	Day 1	Day 2	Day 3	Day 4	Notes
Week 5	Aerobic: 90min CV @ 70% or 90min competitive sport	Strength: 4x 20 press-ups (choice) 4x 20 dips (choice) 4x 20 sit-ups (choice) 4x 45sec core (choice) 4x 20 legs (choice) 4x 8 pull-ups (all at least soldier-level)	Aerobic: 20min CV @ 70% 6x 90sec intervals @ 80% 60sec recovery per rep 6x 45sec intervals @ 80% 30sec recovery per rep	Aerobic / Strength: 60min CV @ 70% 3x 60sec intervals @ 80% 3x 25 press-ups 3x 25 sit-ups 3x 60sec plank (all at least soldier-level)	All interval sessions should be undertaken as an integral activity in the middle of your training session
Week 6	Aerobic: 15min run @ 60% 8x 90sec @ 80% 3min active recovery per rep	Strength: Weights 3x 16 @ 80% shoulders 3x 16 @ 80% triceps 3x 16 @ 80% barbell curl 3x 16 @ 80% chest 3x 16 @ 80% side bend 3x 70sec core (choice) 3x 25 leg circuit ex (choice)	Aerobic: 15min CV @ 60% 5x 60secs @ 90% 3min active recovery per rep	Strength: 4x 22 press-ups (choice) 4x 22 dips (choice) 4x 22 sit-ups (choice) 4x 60sec core (choice) 4x 22 legs (choice) 4x 10 pull-ups (all at least soldier-level)	
Week 7	Aerobic: 40min CV @ 70% 8x 30sec @ 90% Active recovery per rep	Strength: Weights 4x 14 @ 80% shoulders 4x 14 @ 80% triceps 4x 14 @ 80% barbell curl 4x 14 @ 80% chest 4x 14 @ 80% side bend 4x 60sec core (choice) 4x 22 leg circuit ex (choice)	Aerobic: 80min run @ 70% or 90min competitive sport	Aerobic / Strength: 60min CV @ 70% 3x 60sec intervals @ 80% 3x 25 press-ups 3x 25 sit-ups 3x 60sec plank (all at least soldier-level)	
Week 8	Aerobic: 20min run @ 70% 5x 150m hill reps @ 80% Walk down for recovery 5x 100m sprints @ 90% 100m recovery per rep	Strength: 4x 24 press-ups (choice) 4x 24 dips (choice) 4x 24 sit-ups (choice) 4x 70sec core (choice) 4x 24 legs (choice) 4x 12 pull-ups (all at least soldier-level)	Aerobic: 30min CV @ 70% 5x 1min interval @ 90% 30sec recovery per rep	Assessment: Five-Minute Test Middle-distance CV test (choice) BMI Reach Test	Separate CV test and other tests by at least an hour

PERFORMANCE STANDARDS

Cardiovascular Fitness Activity	Civilian	Recruit	Soldier	Paratrooper
Running				
1½ miles	12.31–18 mins	10.30–12.30 mins	8.00–10.31 mins	Under 8 mins
6 miles	51–75 mins	43–50.59 mins	35–42.59 mins	Under 35 mins
10 miles	87–125 mins	75–87 mins	60–75 mins	Under 60 mins
Rowing				
2km	10–15 mins	8–9.59 mins	7–7.59 mins	Under 7 mins
5km	24–32 mins	20–23.59 mins	18–19.59 mins	Under 18 mins
10km	50–70 mins	43–50 mins	39–43 mins	Under 39 mins
Cycling				
20km	45–65 mins	35–44.59 mins	28–34.59 mins	Under 28 mins
40km	90–135 mins	70–89.59 mins	60–69.59 mins	Under 60 mins
80km	180–280 mins	150–179.59 mins	135–149.59 mins	Under 135 mins
Swimming				
750m	20–28 mins	13.30–19.59 mins	11–13.29 mins	Under 11 mins
1500m	45–60 mins	30–44.59 mins	24–29.59 mins	Under 24 mins
3000m	100–135 mins	65–99.59 mins	50–64.59 mins	Under 50 mins
Muscular Endurance	Combined Total Exercises			
Five-Minute Test • Press-ups (1 min) • Sit-ups (1 min) • Star jumps (1 min) • Squat thrusts (1 min) • Burpees (1 min) • 10sec rest between each exercise	0–99	100–199	200–264	Over 265
Flexibility				
Sit & Reach Test (modified version)	30–60cm	20–29.9cm	10–19.9cm	Under 10cm

Achieving paratrooper fitness requires focused preparation and determined effort; use these performance standards to monitor your progress in your preferred activity. The standards have been selected to achieve parity between the exercises. As explained in Part 1, paratrooper fitness blends speed, cardiovascular endurance and muscular endurance. To test your levels in each, on three separate days; attempt the Five-Minute Test, along with the shortest and furthest challenges in your chosen activity (in table above) to see how your fitness levels improves (e.g. if rowing then complete the 2km and 10km in the fastest possible time).

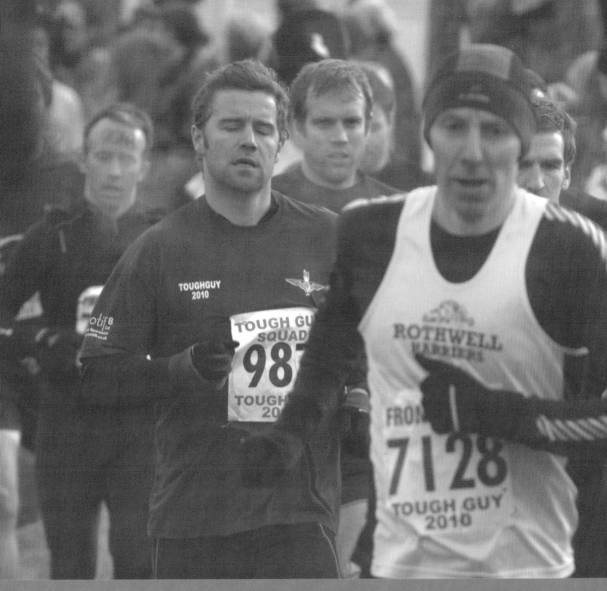

PART 7:
ASPIRATIONAL CHALLENGES

'If my mind can conceive it, and my heart can believe it, I can achieve it.'
Jesse Jackson

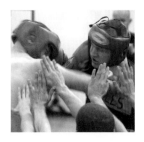

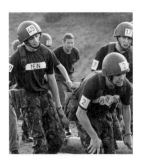

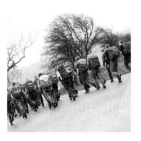

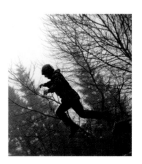

When I addressed students at P Company during my opening speech, I always emphasized that success is determined by mental and physical resilience, but above all else, by the emotional commitment to seeing your chosen activity through to the end. Joining the PARAS is an emotive experience, and unless you are passionate about it the reward is not worth the price. Any physical challenge like P Company pretty soon becomes a mental challenge, and what keeps you going is your commitment and your belief that succeeding in the challenge is worth the punishment you have to put yourself through.

Fitness endeavours and world records are continually being surpassed. However, as the mantra says, 'the race is always against yourself'. I believe people thrive on constant challenge, using incremental steps to break down imaginary walls which stand between them and their potential. Challenges demand a new outlook and approach, and ultimately they cement change and development.

In this book I have tried to give you a means of defining and tackling your goals in a way that makes them more achievable. In this final part, my aim is to encourage you to aspire to things beyond the realm of the PARA fitness programme. Man didn't get to the moon without dreaming of what seemed impossible and taking huge calculated risks. What will your moon be?

In this section, I have purposefully held off giving you the exact training programmes I used to accomplish my fitness goals. You have all the ingredients you need in Parts 2 to 6 to devise your own plan to achieve them and I am certain you will enjoy them all the more when you do. However, I have included insights that you only learn from having done the challenge – particularly where safety is involved.

While you are in the midst of achieving your short-term health and fitness goals, I hope you will read this book and spend some time star-gazing, thinking about what's next. For me it's parenthood, but somewhere on the horizon is my first Iron Man.

Marathons

THE HALF MARATHON

The half marathon is an event that blends long distance with speed. Regardless of your fitness and running ability, it provides a great challenge and training goal. Unlike longer events, the half marathon is easier to train for as both the time and routes to do distance-specific training are easier to find, which is why I believe it is within the grasp of most recreational runners.

What I really like about half marathons is that you get such a broad spectrum of entrants taking part; depending on the profile of the event you can have everyone from Olympic athletes to people wearing deep-sea diver costumes. You can virtually guarantee that you won't come last. Having shown the importance of securing the support of your friends and family (see Part 3), the half marathon is a perfect platform for them to both see the fruits of all your hard training and share in your success. The larger events have an incredibly friendly atmosphere, filled with the family and friends of those taking part.

THE MARATHON

In the half marathon, I would say that the challenge is 80% physical, 20% mental. However, in the marathon these percentages are reversed. The distance of the marathon, both in terms of training and succeeding on race day, makes it more than twice as difficult. To train properly for a marathon requires concerted effort and significantly longer runs in preparation for race day. The distance itself can also form a mental barrier to your success. Expect half-distance in the mental race to be around the 20-mile point and you won't be far wrong. However, while the marathon may be more than twice as difficult as the half marathon, the sense of achievement that comes from completing your first marathon has to be experienced to be believed. During the race, you will fight a constant battle against giving up and it is winning this battle that will give you the most reason for rejoicing at the end. In Part 1, I described the role of P Company as being to sufficiently stretch our recruits so that in the end they realize they are capable of much more than they thought they were – this is what you will get from your first marathon and the only way to experience this empowering feeling is doing it yourself.

ADVICE

There are some things about a marathon and half marathon that you will only learn from doing them. However, the following sections will help you in your preparations.

TRAIN HARD, FIGHT EASY

Remember this mantra? Make sure you have covered a distance at least 80% of your challenge about a month beforehand. This rehearsal is as much about the mental battle as the physical one, and it will condition your mind and body for what lies ahead.

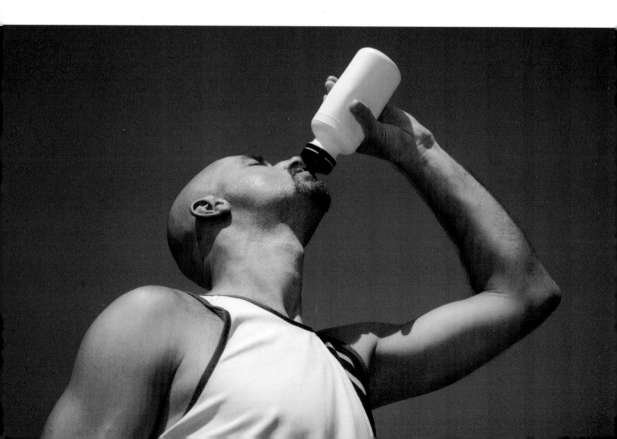

WATER AND FOOD STATIONS

Fuel stations are a common feature of every massed sporting event. As I emphasized in Part 2, remaining hydrated during the race is essential to your success. In the marathon, regular food intake is just as important since your body runs out of carbohydrate stores after two hours of continuous exercise (I am assuming you will be taking more than two hours to complete the race). You need to incorporate eating and drinking while running into your training, as on race day your body will have enough to cope with just completing the race, and having to learn to process food and water for the first time during exercise will be an added burden. As with most things in things in life, less is more. Try to consume small amounts of food and water at every station. What is critical, though, is that you start the race fully hydrated.

MILE MARKERS

Having drummed in the importance of breaking down a challenge into smaller goals, in an organized race much of this is done for you with

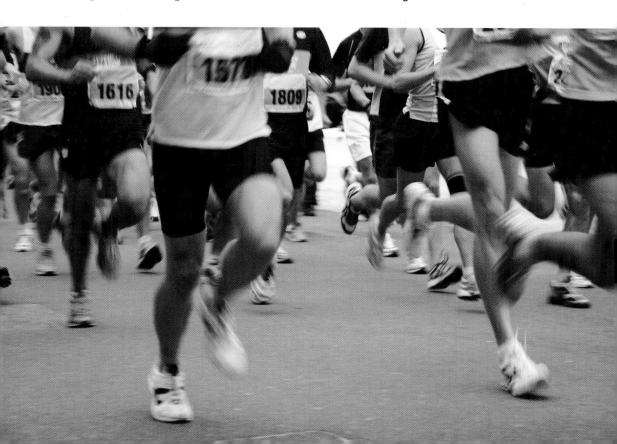

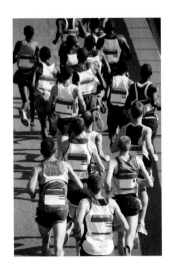

distance markers. Use these markers to your advantage as your short-term focus, but always keep one eye on the finish line. Before you start, have a plan for how long you want to take to do the race, then use that time to work out when you need to be at each marker. This will keep you on track and maintain your focus throughout the race.

MASSED STARTS

Unless you are an elite runner, massed starts are a necessary evil and they will slow you down. You need to prepare for this and factor it into your planning. Plan on not being able to run at your chosen pace for at least the first two miles; how far you are off it will be determined by how many people are running the race. What is important is that you anticipate being behind when you get to your first couple of checkpoints, and you have the chance to think about how you intend to claw your time back without ruining your race by going too quickly when the path clears ahead of you.

RELAX

On the battlefield, much of what happens to us is outside of our control. But in the Parachute Regiment what defines us is how we cope when things go wrong, not when they go to plan. Inevitably, on your first race things won't go to plan, but provided you see the whole thing in the wider context of tackling the most significant fitness challenge of your life, it is possible to win the war even if the battle didn't go the way you'd hoped for. Success is as much about feeling motivated to do another race as it is about smashing your target time.

SHARE YOUR SUCCESS

Training for any significant fitness race such as a half or full marathon can put an incredible strain on your relationships. Invite along all those people who have helped you find the time and motivation to attempt this race and will help you in subsequent challenges. Aside from being the right thing to do, it will maintain their commitment in the future. Why not treat them all at the end to say 'thank you' for their support?

Tough Guy ™

What makes the paratrooper different from the traditional athlete is that in his arena, the game always changes after the starter pistol has been fired. What we are often asked to do for our country is unpleasant and dangerous, but that is what we volunteer for. Before our competition there is no eight hours of undisturbed sleep and no nutritional experts and physios on hand to cater for our every whim. While we can practise every textbook manoeuvre possible, on the day it just won't pan out that way. Our opponents won't play by the rules, while we must. Military training has to replicate these conditions as safely as possible in order to train soldiers for the battlefield. After all, nothing would be more dangerous than a significant gap between what we train for and what we are required to do on the battlefield. This hazardous and uncertain environment is what military training seeks to replicate and so far I haven't found any civilian event better than Tough Guy™ at imitating this.

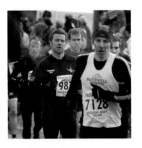

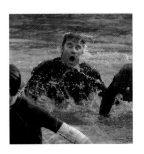

The organizers of Tough Guy somehow manage to deliver a safe event which cuts across modern-day health and safety mollycoddling. Mild hypothermia, black-and-blue limbs and grazed knees are par for the course, which makes the race both deeply unpleasant and retrospectively enjoyable.

Tough Guy is essentially a middle-distance run followed by a long assault course – a description which hides a multitude of pitfalls. Competitors run about six miles before taking on an elaborate assault course that includes 30ft-high climbing frames, tightropes, electric hazards and burning bales of hay. However, by far the most harrowing aspect of Tough Guy is that it's staged in January and you end up being fully immersed in water several times throughout the course. Snow, hail and ice are all commonplace. You arrive at the assault course feeling slightly degraded by the cheeky cross-country course, but you'll arrive at the finish line feeling as though you narrowly avoided death by hypothermia – awesome!

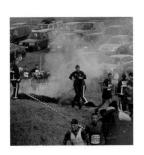

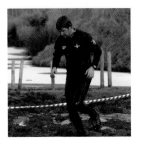

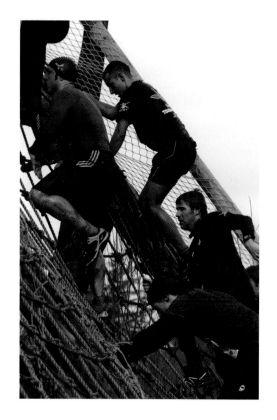

The run has a cult following and regularly attracts upwards of 4,000 competitors. As it is always a mass start, you spend the whole race trying to get as close to the front as possible and trying to avoid freezing while queuing for the next obstacle, by which time it's every man for himself and anything goes.

The race starts out as an aerobic challenge, but evolves into a pseudo-survival situation. There's no doubt it is built on running fitness, but you won't find top-class marathon runners at the front of this event. You need to be fit to get to the assault course in a decent state and preferably ahead of the main pack, but after that it's a test of your resilience and character. If you want to know what it is like to train for eight months to be a paratrooper, this is the best 90-minute insight I've found – you'll want to give up as soon as you get wet.

SPECIALIST KIT REQUIRED

- Running leggings
- Long-sleeved running top
- Fell running/cross-country trainers
- Hat
- Gloves

Bergen Challenges

Although I have included two specific PARA Bergen challenges within this chapter, both based in the UK, it would be very easy for you to create your own P Company-type events. All you really need is a backpack and a suitable route. However, whether you're tackling the PARAS' 10, the Fan Dance, or locally recreating our two-miler, ten-miler or endurance march, here are some tips to make the whole activity as safe and pain-free as possible.

SELECTING A ROUTE

If you are going to create your own P Company test event, you will need to find a route that is both safe and the right distance. I would strongly recommend selecting a route which is predominantly made up of bridleways and is close to roads and civilization in case you get into trouble. Clearly, a potential solution is completing laps of your local park, with a few hill reps thrown in for good measure. However, if you are attempting either the Fan Dance or your own route somewhere off the beaten track here are some tips.

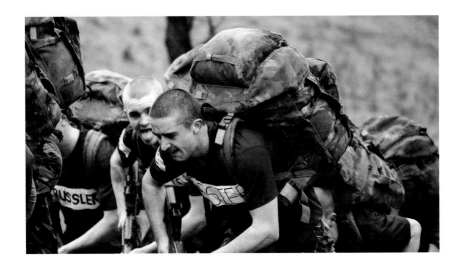

NAVIGATION

Navigation is a critical part of your test. For practical advice on how to map-read go to www.map-reading.com. Thereafter, it is important to have at least studied the route extensively before you set off, ideally using satellite imagery from Google Maps. However, the best possible way to ensure you stay on track during your test day is to recce it beforehand. Remember, time spent on recce is never wasted.

KIT REQUIREMENTS

Depending how off-track you venture here are some items you might need:

- Bergen backpack, ideally with lumbar support and well-padded shoulder straps.
- First aid kit including plasters and zinc oxide tape.
- Waterproof jacket and trousers.
- Sleeping bag and waterproof bivvy bag.
- Warm jumper/jacket or fleece.
- Torch.
- Hat and gloves.
- Mobile phone (for mountain rescue call 999).
- Food and water (as per Part 2).
- Spare socks.
- Well worn-in walking boots (with ankle support).
- Thick socks.
- CamelBak or equivalent water system.
- Map (1:25,000 or 1:50,000).
- Compass.
- GPS – optional and only in addition to a map and compass.

BERGEN PACKING

When packing your Bergen your best bet is to have all your heavy stuff wrapped inside your sleeping bag, as this will reduce the risk of rubbing. After you have packed all essential equipment, weight is best made up with water, which is both useful and quick to dispose of safely if necessary.

LOGISTICAL SUPPORT

When taking on a Bergen challenge, unless you are fortunate enough to have an appropriate testing ground, you will probably need to have some logistical support to make it work. The following is a list of resources which would significantly enhance the safety and enjoyment of your challenge:

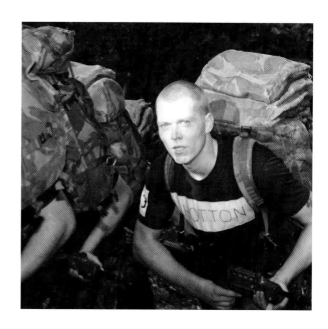

- Vehicle.
- Driver with mobile phone, map and idea of the route, and who knows what to do in the event of a problem.
- Change of clothes.
- Extra food and water for after the challenge.

ABORT CRITERIA

You should abort any Bergen march in the event of the following:

- Snow or ice (present or forecast).
- Wind speed greater than 30mph.
- Temperature either less than 1°C or greater than 20°C.
- Driving rain.
- Thick fog.

ACTIONS ON INJURY

- Stop challenge – inform pre-determined safety person of:
  - Location (8-figure grid reference).
  - Type of injury.
  - Route off the hills.
  - ETA.
- Put on warm kit.

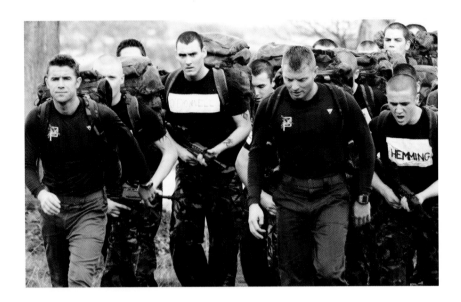

- Treat injury if possible.
- Jettison any water being used for weight purposes, making sure you have sufficient drinking water.
- Make best possible speed to RV.
- Inform safety person when you are off the hills.
- Re-attempt when appropriate.

RECREATING TEST CONDITIONS

Unfortunately, sourcing a dummy weapon will always be a problem and it is not advisable that you try! An extra 10lbs in your Bergen, while considerably less annoying than carrying a long-barrelled weapon, is probably the best option.

P COMPANY TEST EVENTS: KEY INFORMATION

P Company Event/Distance	Height Lost/Gained	Time Allowed
2 miler	650ft	18min
10 miler	2,200ft	1hr 50min
20 miler	4,300ft	4hrs 10 min

The PARAS' 10

The PARAS' 10 is based on the P Company 10-miler described in Part 1. The 10 miler is a core paratrooper test, designed to simulate the move between the parachute drop zone and our objective. The 35lb Bergen simulates a paratrooper's fighting order (the ammunition and equipment carried into battle). As well as being a P Company test event, which all volunteers must pass, it is a weekly feature in PARA battalion life. However, what makes the PARAS' 10 unique as an endurance event is that you effectively do a paratrooper's 10-miler in its entirety; 35lb Bergen, military boots, same route and same time. The cut-off time is one hour 50 minutes. The only thing that differs from the real paratrooper test is the lack of weapons (put in an extra 10lbs if you want), but by tackling it you will get a real sense of whether you have what it takes to pass a PARA test. However, first a word of caution; this is the easy bit, for what follows the 10-miler on the real battlefield is a fight for your life.

The race is staged in September so the weather is normally quite mild, but the Catterick weather has been known to be changeable.

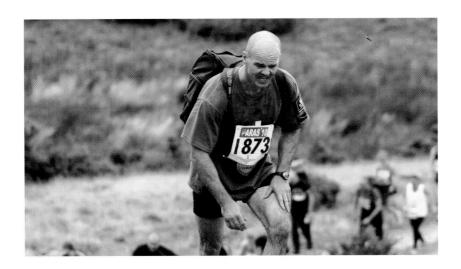

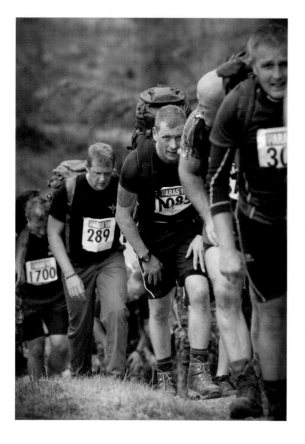

The route is more hilly than mountainous, but it is enclosed entirely within the Catterick military training area, making it much more scenic and exposed than most road runs. However, there are water and first aid stations at the four- and eight-mile points.

On the P Company staff we tackle the 10-miler with monotonous regularity, completing it under test conditions with a course at least every fortnight. I believe tabbing (Tactical Advance to Battle) is picked up easily – all you need is a good base level of fitness, well-fitted boots and a relatively comfy Bergen. The trick is to traverse the ground as efficiently as possible; while some would be capable of running the whole route, your best bet is to stride up the hills and maintain a steady jog on all the flats and the downhill sections. As with any route of moderate distance, it is vital that you maintain your energy and hydration levels.

The added annoyance of heavy boots and an equipment-laden Bergen gives the race a PARA authenticity – one that you will only enjoy after the event, when you're telling your mates about your achievement.

www.paras10.com

The Fan Dance

You could easily be lulled into a false sense of security by the name given to this challenge. However, it is a million miles removed from any musical expression involving Japanese ladies. This Fan Dance is a lung- and thigh-busting 24km march over Pen y Fan, the highest mountain in the Brecon Beacons (2,900ft), which holds legendary status within the British Army. The route is used by many high-profile military units, including 16 Air Assault Brigade's Pathfinder Platoon and the SAS. As a test, the criteria for passing the Fan Dance is identical regardless of who is organizing it; soldiers must complete the course within four hours carrying a 45lb Bergen, a rifle (9lbs) and food and water. The Fan Dance takes a route between the Storey Arms Mountain Rescue Centre

The approach to the top of Pen y Fan, height 2,900ft.

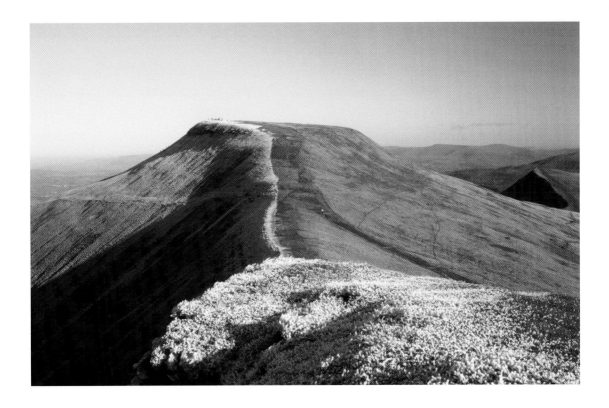

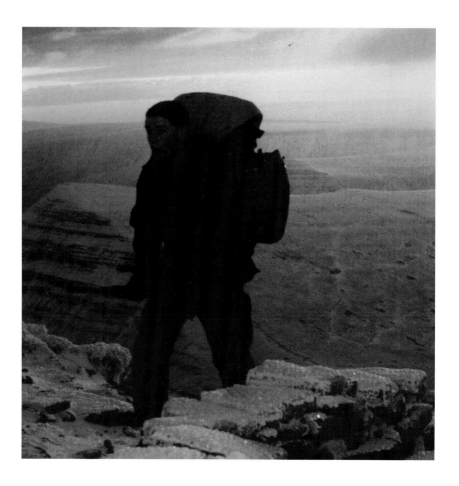

(GR SN 983204) and Torpantau (GR SO 012216), and includes two summits of Pen y Fan.

However, a description of the route undoubtedly hide the fiery breath and teeth of this Welsh dragon. Over the years, I've done this route in many guises and it has always been emotional. Do it in a group under four hours and it will always end in an orgy of self-congratulation! Don't be put off by the headlines; in my opinion getting around this route in four hours is closer to half marathon rather than marathon levels of difficulty – assuming that you're running at the crest of your ability rather than just ahead of the pantomime horse. The trick, as ever, is focused training and preparation, with a bit of good luck thrown in.

As you would expect from a route used to select some of our A-team, the terrain is unforgiving by design. That said, navigation (on a clear day)

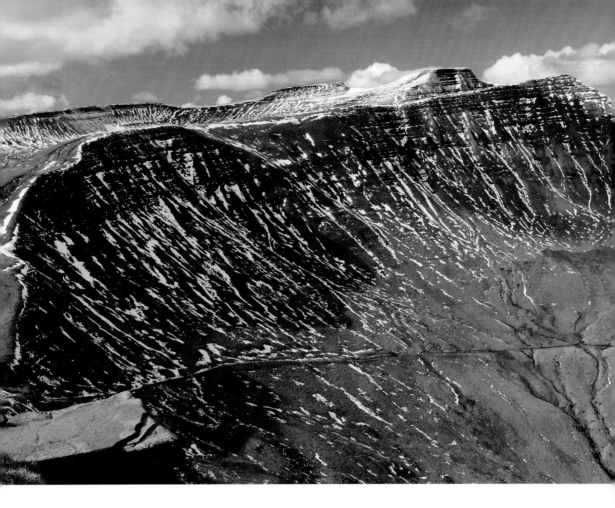

is relatively simple as the route is entirely over footpaths and bridleways. Inevitably, what makes a tough challenge impossible is the weather, which unfortunately on a number of occasions has proved fatal. Safety on anything as demanding as the Fan Dance can never be guaranteed, but serious injury can be avoided by working within your limits, respecting the weather, and carrying appropriate safety equipment. Unlike the previous challenges, this is an event you can recreate at a time and date of your own choosing. It requires much more planning and logistics than a staged fitness event and, unless you live in Brecon, this will be a much more expensive challenge than those described above. However, the confidence that comes from knowing you have completed it within the cut-off time is well worth the premium. Unlike the other challenges, the Fan Dance doesn't include crowds of well-wishers, nor are there medals, T-shirts, and an official time at the finish, but then solitary achievements have their own rewards, which nourish the soul rather than the ego.

The Bob Graham Round – A Quantum Leap!

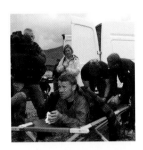

The Bob Graham Round is a 42-mountain, 72-mile circuit in England's Lake District and includes 27,000ft of vertical ascent (equivalent to Everest). The round is named after Bob Graham (1889–1966), a Keswick guest-house owner, who in 1932 on his 42nd birthday set the record for the number of Lakeland fells (42) traversed in 24 hours. Any contender who traverses the Bob Graham fells within 24 hours is eligible for membership of the Bob Graham Club. It is considered by many, including Everest adventurer Chris Bonnington, as one of the most elite endurance clubs in the world. Since 1932, only 1,500 people have joined the club. However, the spirit of the club, derived from its founder, is far from elitist and its aim is simply to support, encourage and record new members on their attempts.

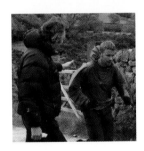

My motive for attempting and completing the Bob Graham Round in 2009 came from my work colleagues. As a serving paratrooper, I have seen many of my friends killed and seriously injured on operations. On New Year's Day 2009 I decided that I would do something to raise money for Help for Heroes, a charity that has helped my friends, colleagues and their dependants in some of their darkest moments. Out of respect for both the people I was raising money for and those whom I was asking to donate, I wanted to tackle a challenge that would test all of my resources: the Bob Graham Round. The idea of attempting the Bob Graham Round came to me nearly 12 years ago, after noticing a picture of legendary fell runner Joss Naylor on a Bob Graham Round while I was drinking a pint in the Wasdale Head Inn after having run up Scafell Pike. In an instant, running up the highest mountain in England went from impressive to insignificant!

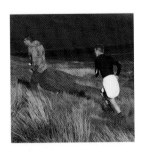

I recruited a close friend, and fellow paratrooper, to attempt the Bob Graham Round and over the next five months, we spent alternate weekends training, recceing and planning for our round. As neither of us were members of a fell running club, we knew that we wouldn't be

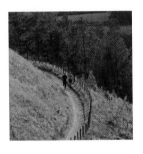

able to call on experienced pacers on the day and undertook to know the route inside-out before our attempt. With the exception of an ex-paratrooper, Derek Eland, who looked after our roadside support, we were supported by a group of novice fell runners, drawn from friends within the Parachute Regiment.

We started our round at 1900hrs on Saturday 6 June; the 65th anniversary of the Parachute Regiment's Battle of Normandy. Despite some pretty horrendous weather during the previous 24 hours, when we set off the conditions were dry and cool – perfect for our attempt. After Skiddaw, my friend and I had to tackle Great Calva and Blencathra alone as our pacers struggled to keep up, but we got to the first checkpoint in Threlkeld nearly ten minutes ahead of our 22-hour schedule.

The next section to Dunmail Rise proved to be hideous; the visibility was less than five metres, and there were gale force winds and snow on the summits – so much for it being summer! During the second leg, my running partner became violently sick and gradually became slower and more incoherent. We got to Dunmail nearly two hours over our schedule and spirits were very low.

During the third section, I was on my own and had to put everything I had into clawing back some of my lost time. Fortunately, two climber friends – Bruce, a former OC P Company, and Jacko, my CO – volunteered to rope me up Broad Stand, a treacherous short-cut that saved me at least 20 minutes, which later proved vital. I arrived at Wasdale physically and emotionally drained, but more importantly back on track to complete the round within 24 hours.

Outside the Moot Hall, Keswick High Street – the start and finish point of the legendary Bob Graham Round circuit.

By the fourth leg, I was running on willpower rather than fitness, but tackled the hills almost on pace with my close friend Brian, and his dog Phoebe (who made the

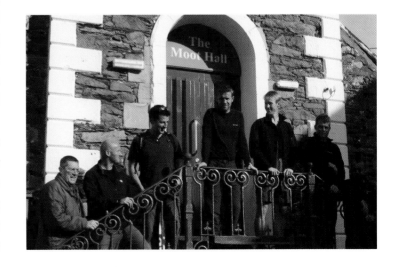

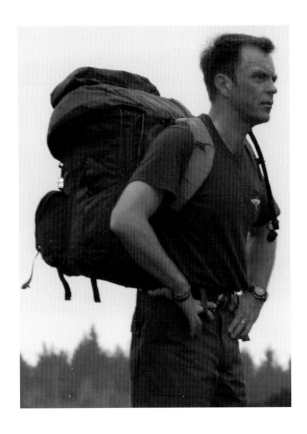

Lt Col Andy Jackson (my former CO), who led me up Broad Stand with Bruce Radbourne during my Bob Graham Round.

section look easy). At Honister, the round was looking very achievable, and nearly 30 supporters were there to encourage me before my final leg. Over the next three hills, accompanied by nearly a section of paratroopers, I felt my body getting gradually wearier, but nothing was going to stop me from banging the Moot Hall door within 24 hours of my start. My wife Annie ran and walked the final road section with me, which was a fitting way to conclude a challenge that had been the focus of the last six months of my life, and had had a heavy impact on her life too. Despite much bravado in the days leading up to my attempt, I decided to pass on a pint at the Swinside Inn. I managed a sprint up Keswick High Street, just beating my Dad, and hit the Moot Hall door with a little over 15 minutes to spare. Elated, emotional and completely shattered, in 23 hours 45 minutes, we had raised over £7,000 for Help for Heroes; nearly a pound for every mile!

As my attempt was the feature of a BBC1 documentary, I can say what I said in the interview prior to my Bob Graham Round without fear of being called a liar. At no time throughout my training and attempt did I ever doubt that I would succeed. I could attribute my confidence to many things, but above all else there is one I would urge you to imitate. For six months I had spent a great deal of time thinking about myself running over the 42 mountains, but in particular thinking about what I would see, hear and feel when I crossed the finish line inside 24 hours. Even as I write this, a wave of emotion comes over me. The sense of elation that I got from visualising an experience which hadn't even taken place was an incredibly potent motivator. In January, that visualisation was my destination, but what fuelled the journey for the next six months was the love and support of my wife, family and friends.

APPENDICES:

GLOSSARY OF MAJOR MUSCLE GROUPS

FRONT

Biceps

These muscles run across the front of each arm between the shoulder and elbows.

Deltoids

These muscles surround the fleshy part of the shoulder.

Pectorals

These muscles span the chest.

Rectus abdominals

These muscles stem from the bottom of the rib cage to the top of the legs.

Hip flexors

These muscles bridge the gap between the thighs and the waist.

Quadraceps

These muscles span between the top of the leg and the knee.

BACK

Rhomboid and trapezius

These muscles are between the middle of the back and the shoulders.

Latissimus dorsi

These muscles span the lower three-quarters of the back from roughly below the shoulders.

Triceps

These muscles stretch between the elbow and shoulder on the back of the arm.

Quadratus lumborum

These muscles sit at the rear and side of the waist.

Gluteals

These muscles form the bottom and hips.

Hamstrings

These muscles stretch between the top of the back of the leg and the knee.

Calves

These muscles span between the heel and knee and the back of the leg.

TABLES AND EXERCISE SHEETS

REPORTING FOR DUTY STANDARD

Starting Fitness Level

Activity	ASSESSMENT SCORE	PERFORMANCE STANDARDS			
		Civilian	Recruit	Soldier	Paratrooper
Pull-ups		0–5	6–10	11–17	18 or more
Press-ups (2mins)		0–29	30–49	50–79	80 or more
Sit-ups (2mins)		0–29	30–49	50–79	80 or more
1½-mile run		12.31–18min	10.31–12.30min	8.01–10.30min	Under 8min
Reach Test		60–31cm	30–21cm	11–20cm	Under 10cm
BMI		30–39.9	25–29.9	18.5–24.9	Under 18.5
Resting heart rate		80–110	65–80	50–65	Under 50

What you want to achieve?

Specific	
Measureable	
Achievable Do you have the sufficient time, knowledge, skills and physical resources to achieve this?	
Relevant Is this relevant to your wider goal?	
Time-specific	

Why you will succeed?

WORK TOWARDS YOUR GOAL		DO NOTHING	
Pleasure	Pain	Pleasure	Pain

	Day 1	Day 2	Day 3	Day 4	Notes
Week 1	Session goal:	Session goal:	Session goal:	Session goal:	
Week 2	Session goal:	Session goal:	Session goal:	Session goal:	
Week 3	Session goal:	Session goal:	Session goal:	Session goal:	
Week 4	Session goal:	Session goal:	Session goal:	Session goal:	

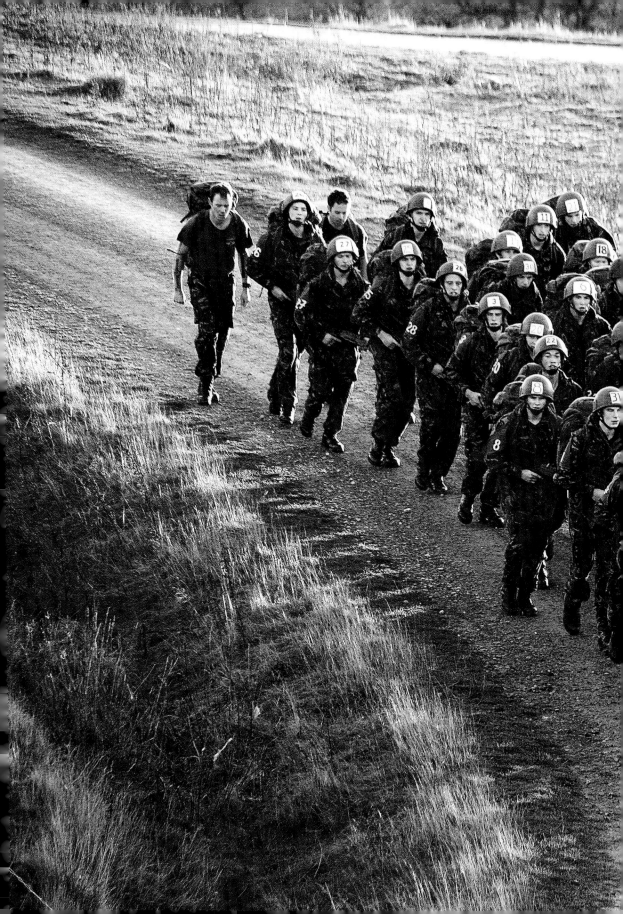

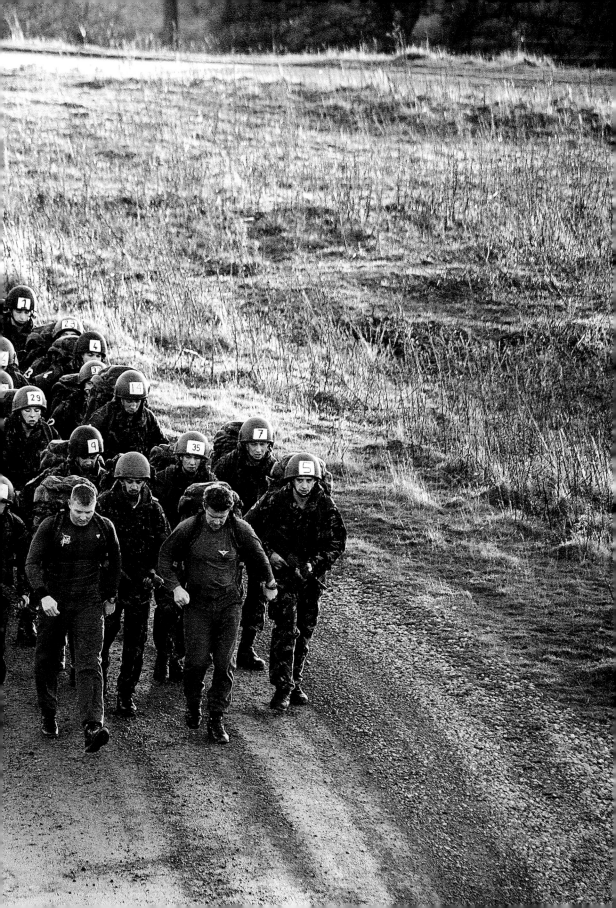

FINDING TIME: YOUR FITNESS TRAINING BATTLE PLAN

	0100	0300	0500	0700	0900	11
Monday						
Tuesday						
Wednesday						
Thursday						
Friday						
Saturday						
Sunday						

	Sleep	Work on maintaining at least seven hours, if anything you will need more when you are exercising.
	Work/College	Is there scope to train on your way to or from work/college or during your lunch break?
	Commitments	Any event which is important to you or your family and friends.
	Potential Pitfalls	These are events or potential events that could either stop you from training or eliminate the benefit you are getting from training.
	Opportunities	Free time to train.
	Fuel	Put your food in last, unless it is a social occasion. You should aim to plan your diet around your activities. For guidance see page 56.

Objective: Fill a time line of your typical week in order to identify:
1. Suitable windows for training – exploit.
2. Events which have the ability to cannibalise your fitness goal – avoid.

Critical Success Factors?
1. Time: How long do I need for each training session? (Include travel and changing time.)
2. Resources: What space, equipment do I need before or after my session? (Sports kit, spare work clothes, shower, food etc.)
3. Fuel: How do I need to manage where, when and what I eat in order to be able to train?
4. Win-Win: How do I score a double victory, replacing a potential pitfall with a training session?
5. Redundancy: Where can I find additional sessions if I need to?
6. Friendly Forces: Whose help do I need to secure to be able to achieve my goal and how can I sell it to them?
7. Enemies: Who, where and what do I need to avoid in order to guarantee success?

1300				1500				1700				1900				2100				2300			

CREDITS

The author and publishers are grateful to those below for permission to include images:

Anthony Thomas (www.euroshots.com); p.181

Boundford.com; p.64

Channelle Knapp (www.elegance-photography.co.uk); back cover (top right), p.5, pp.8–9, p.12, p.14, pp.20–24
(all images), pp.26–27 (all images), p.46, p.57, pp.69–70 (all images), p.76, pp.98–99
(all images), p.102–103, p.166 (all images), p.173, pp.175–176 (all images) and pp.188–189

Claudia Janke; p.7 (left)

Corbis; p.67 (second down) and p.179

Gareth Netherwood; p.180

Gary Evans (www.myeventphoto.co.uk); pp.177–178 (all images)

Getty Images; back cover (top centre), p.10, p.16, p.17, pp.30–32 (background image), pp.62–
64 (background image), p.67 (top, third and fourth down), pp.79–80 (background image), p.82,
pp.94–96 (background image), pp.137–138 (background image), p.137 and p.138

Imperial War Museum; p.30 (courtesy of the Lord Ashcroft collection), p.62 (H17365),
p.94 (FKD41) and p.95 (FKD851)

Istock; p.54, p.73, p.147, p.149, p.150 and pp.168–170 (all images)

Ken Ford; p.63, p.79 and p.80

Colonel Lee Walters; p.66

Martin Hothersall; pp.182–183 (all images)

Matt Timbers (www.matttimbers.com); front cover, back cover (top left), back flap, p.6, p.11,
p.13, p.15, pp.28–29 (all images), pp.33–45 (all images), p.47, p.49, p.51, p.53, p.59, p.61, p.65,
p.75 (all images), p.81, pp.83–93 (all images), p.97, p.101, pp.104–125 (all images), p.128,
p.135 (both images), pp.139–146 (all images), p.141, pp.151–157 (all images), p.165 and
pp.171–172 (all images)

Ministry of Defence; p.30

Major Sam McGrath; p.148

Soldier Magazine; p.18, p.25 (both images) and p.71

The Afghanistan Trust; p.7 (right)